INTRODUCTION
EBDM in Action: Developing Competence in Evidence-Based Practice
FOUNDATION FOR EVIDENCE-BASED DECISION MAKING

Evidence-based Decision Making (EBDM) is the formalized process of using the skills for identifying, searching for and interpreting the results of the best scientific evidence which is considered in conjunction with the clinician's experience and judgment, the patient's preferences and values, and the clinical/patient circumstances when making patient care decisions. We view EBDM as a tool to improve the quality of care and to reduce the gap between what we know and what we do.

EBDM in Action: Developing Competence in Evidence-Based Practice teaches the critical thinking skills necessary for life-long learning and providing evidence-based patient care. Each module integrates and builds upon the 5 skills of the evidence-based process.

Skill 1. ASK: Converting Information Needs/Problems Into Clinical Questions So That They Can Be Answered

Skill 2. ACCESS: Conducting A Computerized Search With Maximum Efficiency For Finding the Best External Evidence with which to Answer the Question

Skill 3. APPRAISE: Critically Appraising the Evidence for its Validity and Usefulness

Skill 4. APPLY: Applying the Results of the Appraisal, or Evidence, In Clinical Practice

Skill 5. ASSESS: Evaluating the Process and your Performance

This book reflects over two decades of cumulative experience designing educational materials, facilitating workshops and educating health professionals on how to integrate the evidence-based process into practice. It presents content based on each skill including formulating patient-centered questions, searching for the appropriate evidence, critically appraising the evidence, applying the evidence to practice, and evaluating the process.

EBDM in Action focuses on the Continuum of Competence - Novice, Beginner, and Competent so that learners acquire evidence-based skills. Fill-in, multiple choice and online assignments help solidify the beginning steps necessary to become a critical thinker. The learner should move from just knowing to applying previous knowledge, assessing research for its relevancy and knowing when to apply it.

Each chapter identifies the related CODA standards or relevant portions thereof, has specific objectives and contains suggested assignments including critical thinking and self-reflection questions and exercises to reinforce learning. As readers progresses through each chapter, assignments and assessments can be used to document their progress. This demonstrates learning and applying the EBDM process and skills related to answering patient questions about therapy/prevention, diagnosis, etiology/harm/causation and prognosis.

ACCREDITATION STANDARDS FOR DENTAL EDUCATION PROGRAMS

Commission on Dental Accreditation
211 East Chicago Ave.
Chicago, Illinois 60611

EDUCATIONAL ENVIRONMENT

Critical Thinking

Critical thinking is foundational to teaching and deep learning in any subject. The components of critical thinking are: the application of logic and accepted intellectual standards to reasoning; the ability to access and evaluate evidence; the application of knowledge in clinical reasoning; and a disposition for inquiry that includes openness, self-assessment, curiosity, skepticism, and dialogue. In professional practice, critical thinking enables the dentist to recognize pertinent information, make appropriate decisions based on a deliberate and open-minded review of the available options, evaluate outcomes of diagnostic and therapeutic decisions, and assess his or her own performance. Accordingly, the dental educational program must develop students who are able to:

- Identify problems and formulate questions clearly and precisely;
- Gather and assess relevant information, weighing it against extant knowledge and ideas, to interpret information accurately and arrive at well-reasoned conclusions;
- Test emerging hypotheses against evidence, criteria, and standards;
- Show intellectual breadth by thinking with an open mind, recognizing and evaluating assumptions, implications, and consequences;
- Communicate effectively with others while reasoning through problems.

Evidence-based Care

Evidence-based dentistry (EBD) is an approach to oral health care that requires the judicious integration of systematic assessments of clinically relevant scientific evidence, relating to the patient's oral and medical condition and history, with the dentist's clinical expertise and the patient's treatment needs and preferences. EBD uses thorough, unbiased systematic reviews and critical appraisal of the best available scientific evidence in combination with clinical and patient factorsto make informed decisions about appropriate health care for specific clinical cirmcumstances.

Scientific Discovery and the Integration of Knowledge

The interrelationship between the basic, behavioral, and clinical sciences is a conceptual cornerstone to clinical competence. Learning must occur in the context of real health care problems rather than within singular content-specific disciplines. Learning objectives that cut across traditional disciplines and correlate with the expected competencies of graduates enhance curriculum design. Beyond the acquisition of scientific knowledge at a particular point in time, the capacity to think scientifically and to apply the scientific method is critical if students are to analyze and solve oral health problems, understand research, and practice evidence-based dentistry.

EBDM IN ACTION:
Developing Competence in EB Practice

Jane L. Forrest, EdD, RDH

Director,
National Center for Dental Hygiene Research & Practice, Inc.
Cave Creek, AZ

Professor Emerita,
Herman Ostrow School of Dentistry of University of Southern California
Los Angeles, CA

Syrene A. Miller, BA

Project Manager,
National Center for Dental Hygiene Research & Practice, Inc.
Spokane, WA

EBDMinACTION.com
Cave Creek, AZ

Second Edition
Copyright ©2020 JL Forrest & SA Miller

EBDM in ACTION
PO BOX 4348
Cave Creek, AZ 85327

Printed in the United States

Library of Congress Cataloging-In-Publication Data

Evidence-based Decision-making in Action: Developing Competence in Evidence Based Practice
Jane L. Forrest and Syrene A. Miller
Includes bibliographical references
ISBN-10: 0-9974121-2-7
ISBN-13: 978-0-9974121-2-3

1. Evidence-based dentistry. 2. Dentistry-Decision making. 3. Clinical Decision-Making. 4. Developing Competency

Care has been taken to confirm the accuracy of the information presented and to describe generally accepted practices. However, the authors / editors / and publisher are not responsible for errors or omissions or for any consequences from application of the information in this book and make no warranty, expressed or implied, with respect to the currency, completeness, or accuracy of the contents of the publication. Application of this information in a particular situation remains the professional responsibility of the practitioner; the clinical treatments described and recommended may not be considered absolute and universal recommendations.

The authors, editors, and publisher have exerted every effort to ensure that drug selection and dosage set forth in this text in accordance with the current recommendation and practice at the time of publication. However, in view of ongoing research, changes in government regulations and the constant flow of information relating to drug therapy and drug reactions, the reader is urged to check the package insert for each drug for any change in indications and dosage and for added warnings and precautions. This is particularly important when the recommended agent is a new or infrequently employed drug.

Some drugs and medical devices presented in this publication have Food Drug Administration (FDA) clearance for limited use in restricted research settings. It is the responsibility of the health care provider to ascertain the FDA status of each drug or device planned for use in their clinical practice.

To purchase copies of this book, visit EBDM in ACTION: http://ebdminaction.com or email jforrest@ebdminaction.com

STANDARD 2 - EDUCATIONAL PROGRAM

Critical Thinking

2- 10 Graduates **must** be competent in the use of critical thinking and problem-solving, including their use in the comprehensive care of patients, scientific inquiry and research methodology.

Intent: Throughout the curriculum, the educational program should use teaching and learning methods that support the development of critical thinking and problem solving skills

Self-Assessment

2-11 Graduates **must** demonstrate the ability to self-assess, including the development of professional competencies and the demonstration of professional values and capacities associated with self-directed, lifelong learning.

Intent: Educational program should prepare students to assume responsibility for their own learning. The education program should teach students how to learn and apply evolving and new knowledge over a complete career as a health care professional. Lifelong learning skills include student assessment of learning needs.

Clinical Sciences

2-22 Graduates **must** be competent to access, critically appraise, apply, and communicate scientific and lay literature as it relates to providing evidence-based patient care.

Intent:
The education program should introduce students to the basic principles of clinical and translational research, including how such research is conducted, evaluated, applied, and explained to patients.

STANDARD 5 - PATIENT CARE SERVICES

5-2 Patient care **must** be evidenced-based, integrating the best research evidence and patient values.

Intent:
The dental school should use evidence to evaluate new technology and products and to guide diagnosis and treatment decisions.

ACCREDITATION STANDARDS FOR DENTAL HYGIENE EDUCATION PROGRAMS

Commission on Dental Accreditation
211 East Chicago Ave.
Chicago, Illinois 60611

Copyright © 2018,
Commission on Dental
Accreditation

312/440-4653
www.ada.org/coda
Effective January 1, 2013

PATIENT CARE COMPETENCIES

2-13 Graduates must be competent in providing the dental hygiene process of care, which includes:

d) provision of patient-centered treatment and evidence-based care in a manner minimizing risk and optimizing oral health;

Examples of evidence to demonstrate compliance may include:
- Evidence-based treatment strategies

CRITICAL THINKING

2-21 Graduates must be competent in the application of self-assessment skills to prepare them for life-long learning.

Intent:
Dental hygienists should possess self-assessment skills as a foundation for maintaining competency and quality assurance.
Examples of evidence to demonstrate compliance may include:
- Written course documentation of content in self-assessment skills
- Evaluation mechanisms designed to monitor knowledge and performance
- Outcomes assessment mechanisms

2-22 Graduates must be competent in the evaluation of current scientific literature.

Intent:
Dental hygienists should be able to evaluate scientific literature as a basis for life-long learning, evidenced-based practice and as a foundation for adapting to changes in healthcare.
Examples of evidence to demonstrate compliance may include:
- Written course documentation of content in the evaluation of current and classic scientific literature
- Evaluation mechanisms designed to monitor knowledge and performance
- Outcomes assessment mechanisms

2-23 Graduates must be competent in problem solving strategies related to comprehensive patient care and management of patients.

Intent:
Critical thinking and decision-making skills are necessary to provide effective and efficient dental hygiene services. Throughout the curriculum, the educational program should use teaching and learning methods that support the development of critical thinking and problem solving skills.
Examples of evidence to demonstrate compliance may include:
- Evaluation mechanisms designed to monitor knowledge and
- performance;
- Outcomes assessment mechanisms demonstrating application of critical thinking skills;
- Activities or projects that demonstrate student experiences with analysis of problems related to comprehensive patient care;
- Demonstration of the use of active learning methods that promote critical appraisal of scientific evidence in combination with clinical application and patient factors.

I

FOUNDATION FOR EVIDENCE-BASED DECISION MAKING

STAGE OF COMPETENCY - NOVICE: KNOWS

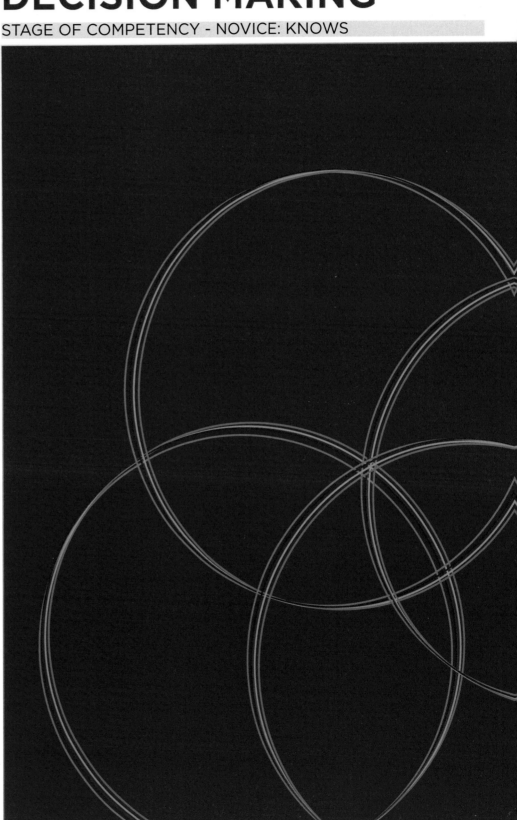

CHAPTER

1

BECOMING A COMPETENT EVIDENCE-BASED PRACTITIONER

Skill 5: Evaluating the process and your performance

Content Outline:
Continuum of Competence
Documenting Competence
   Development
Conclusion
Assignments
References

Learning Objectives:
Upon completion of this chapter,
1. Understand how the continuum of competence illustrates the process of becoming a competent practitioner
2. Understand how assessment tools will be used to evaluate performance in developing EBDM skills.
3. Identify additional learning needs and strategies based on results from self-reflection and self-assessments.

Suggested Assignments:
Baseline Assessment
Critical Thinking Questions
Self-Reflection Questions

The purpose of this chapter is to introduce the self-assessment and evaluation methods used throughout this book. Mastering the skills of evidence based decision-making (EBDM) takes practice and reflection. Encountering early difficulties should not discourage a clinician who is new to this process. Educational rubrics and developing a personal EB portfolio are helpful tools in the development of EBDM skills and the integration of scientific evidence into everyday practice to improve patient care and outcomes.

DDS/DMD CODA STANDARDS
EDUCATIONAL ENVIRONMENT, Critical Thinking: The components of critical thinking are: ...the application of knowledge in clinical reasoning; and a disposition for inquiry that includes openness, self-assessment ... In professional practice, critical thinking enables the dentist to... evaluate outcomes of diagnostic and therapeutic decisions, and assess his or her own performance. Accordingly, students must be able to: Recognize and evaluate assumptions, implications, and consequences

Self-Assessment, 2-11 Graduates must demonstrate the ability to self-assess, including the development of professional competencies and the demonstration of professional values and capacities associated with self-directed, lifelong learning.

DH CODA STANDARDS
Critical Thinking, 2-21: Graduates must be competent in the application of self-assessment skills to prepare them for life-long learning.
Intent: Dental hygienists should possess self-assessment skills as a foundation for maintaining competency and quality assurance.

CONTINUUM OF COMPETENCE

New CODA standards require the development of:
Critical Thinking
Evidence-Based Patient Care
Life-long learning using evidence-based principles
Self-assessment skills
Principles of clinical and translational research
Knowledge of how research is conducted, evaluated, applied, and explained to patients

Miller's Pyramid of Clinical Competence, has gained acceptance in professional education.[1] The continuum includes 5 stages (Figure 1-1) beginning with novice, and then proceeding through the stages of beginner, competent, proficient and culminating with expert.[2] Students in professional education enter at the novice stage and through a series of learning experiences progress to towards achieving competence by the time they graduate. The dental/dental hygiene educational curriculum must demonstrate that graduates have developed competence, leaving the development of proficiency and expertise for later.[3,4]

Expertise develops over time with practice experiences and reflection. The five developmental stages of competence also can be applied to the development of EBDM skills.

1. A **Novice** learner requires educational opportunities to learn theory and rules and needs frequent guidance and evaluation. It is based on developing cognition through fact gathering and is built around the cognition zone **Knows**.

2. At the **Beginner** level of the learning curve, students can understand theory but cannot always connect it to practice. It states the learner **Knows How** and can interpret and apply knowledge through case presentations and essays, but still needs direction to guide behavior.

3. At the **Competent** level students can integrate theory with practice and demonstrate the abilities of EBDM **without help**. Under this category a student **Shows** by demonstrating their learning using behavior that is independent of direction from faculty.

4. **Proficient** practitioners can combine analytical thinking with intuitive experience with greater depth and breadth of understanding in a wide range of cases, **Does.**

5. The final phase on the continuum is **Expert**, which involves effortlessly completing the EBDM process and easily incorporating each aspect into everyday practice while blending the highest level of judgment and skills. Table 1-1 compares the behaviors of a student at each level of the continuum.

Figure 1-1 Continuum of Competence

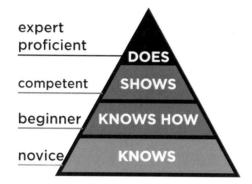

expert
proficient
DOES
competent
SHOWS
beginner
KNOWS HOW
novice
KNOWS

Effortlessly & intuitively incorporates EBDM in to everyday practice.

Integrates theory with practice and demonstrates the EBDM skills and process independently.

Understands theory but can not always connect it to practice. Still needs guidance.

Requires educational opportunities to learn theory, skills, aspects of the evidence-based process. Needs frequent guidance and evaluation to develop comprehension.

Table 1-1 Behaviors during Problem Solving[5]				
Novice: Knows	**Beginner: Knows How**	**Competent: Shows**	**Proficient: Does**	**Expert: Does**
Slow Just learning	Hesitant	Analytical & Deliberate	Greater Breadth & Depth of Understanding	Fast and fluid
Requires lecture and labs to learn theory, and rules	Requires practice in multiple applications with varying situations	Demonstrates basic abilities of a safe, independent practitioner	Demonstrates abilities with a wide range of situations	Uses intuition and experience without conscious analytic thinking
Lacks full understanding	Understands theory and rules, but cannot always connect it to clinical situations	Integrates theory and practice. Has a variety of possible solutions to problems.	Provides leadership even when situation is ambiguous and outcome is uncertain	Effortlessly completes tasks as normal
Requires frequent guidance and needs to learn theory and rules	Requires practice using a variety of situations. Still requires feedback. Rule bound; tries to implement textbook approaches	Can complete the process independently without feedback. Ability to discern pertinent information	Adapts to circumstances; not locked into any one particular strategy. Mixes analytical thinking with intuitive experience.	Blends highest level of judgment and skill
Externally Motivated	"Trial and error" efforts to solve the problem using one approach at a time	Able to independently implement a course of action	Settles on the "best course of action" after quick review of options but willing to change course if results are not satisfactory	Is able to combine all decision making skills to solve a problem with little effort

* Adapted from Hendrickson, et al. 2006[5]

The learning curve for many aspects of EBDM is quite steep. However, with time and practice, the climb towards becoming an expert evidence-based practitioner is easily within reach. Identifying learning needs based on self-reflection assignments and self-assessment can aid in improving performance. Reviewing the related chapters can strengthen the weak areas. Additional tutorials and resources are available on the website, ebdLibrary.com, which has valuable resources related to each aspect of the EBDM process.

DOCUMENTING COMPETENCE DEVELOPMENT

Portfolios in dental and dental hygiene education can be used to document and evaluate the development of competence in many areas, including evidence-based decision making. (EBDM) Portfolio learning is an assessment method that encourages reflective learning and facilitates the collection of evidence and educational experiences over time that document learning has taken place.[6,7] It allows students and faculty to monitor performance and the practical application of theory. Portfolio learning also can encourage professional and personal growth by stimulating learning that can impact behavior, perception and performance. Activities in this book have been designed to allow students to document their growth in the EBDM process culminating in their demonstration of competency, as per the ADA CODA standards regarding evidence-based dentistry, critical thinking and self-assessment.

SELF-REFLECTION

Reflecting on each step of the process of EBDM and evaluating performance is necessary to build EBDM skills. Each chapter contains self-reflection questions that provide learners an opportunity to find meaning in their learning.   Reflective questioning prompts learners to expand their thinking and document changes in thinking and how they respond to their educational experiences.

SELF-ASSESSMENT

In addition to the Critical Thinking and Self-Reflection questions at the end of each chapter, there are two different assessment tools, or rubrics for student use. These can be used by students to monitor their skill development progress and to understand what is expected.

1. The **EBDM in Action Self-Assessment** rubric accompanies every chapter, specific to each skill in the evidence-based process (Table 1-2). This tool is based on the Continuum of Competence, Novice through Proficient (Figure 1-1, Table 1-1). The expectation of students during this process is based on achieving EBDM skills at the Competent level by the time of graduation. The rubric includes the Proficient level to identify a detailed target for student to strive towards regarding incorporating EBDM into practice. The Expert level requires time, practice and experience to develop skills that easily flow and are seamlessly integrated into everyday practice. This level is not realistic during to achieve in an educational program.

    The rubric clearly delineates the expectations of the skills for the PICO process, completing a computerized search, critically appraising the research, and applying the appraisal results in clinical practice. Students can use them for self-assessment and self-correction prior to turning in an assignment that will be graded by the instructor. In addition, these rubrics can be used for peer evaluation related to each of the skill areas. An example of the EBDM in Action Self-Assessment rubric for skill 1 is provided in Table 1-2. The complete rubric can be found in the resources section.

Rubrics for learning:

A scoring rubric is designed to communicate clear expectations, consistent grading criteria and fair assessment of the quality of students' work especially when responses can be subjective or complex.

Rubrics create a basis for self-evaluation, reflection, and peer review. They cultivate understanding, and encourage learning by providing definitive standards at different levels of achievement.[8]

Table 1-2 EBDM in Action Self-Assessment

Skill 5. ASSESS: Evaluating The Process And Your Performance

Rate your performance of each aspect of EBDM by identifying where you are on the competence continuum. Outline how you plan to strengthen your weaknesses in the comments section.

PICO PROCESS

Skill 1. ASK: Converting Problems Into Clinical Questions So That They Can Be Answered

Novice (Knows)	Beginner (Knows How)	Competent (Shows How)	Proficient (Does)
Just learning, lacks full understanding, and needs to learn theory and rules. **Requires frequent guidance and feedback.**	Understands the theory and rules, but can't completely demonstrate the process; requires practice using a variety of situations. **Still requires feedback.**	Demonstrates basic abilities of EBDM; integrates theory and practice; has variety of possible solutions to problems; can complete the process **independently without feedback.**	Greater depth and breadth of understanding and demonstrates abilities with a wide range of cases; adapts to circumstances and willing to change if results are not satisfactory. Mixes analytical thinking with intuitive experience.

Rate ability based on competence level:	Novice Just Learning	Beginner Requires Practice	Competent Highly Capable	Proficient Expertly Skilled
Question is clearly focused, stated in the correct format, and effectively outlines the problem using; only relevant descriptor(s), a well-defined intervention, a precise comparison and measurable outcome(s) that clearly addresses the problem or patient.				
Problem or patient population is carefully delineated and description is as specific as needed (patient population, sub-group, sex, ethnicity, setting of interest, disease/ condition/ disorder). Irrelevant descriptors are not included.				
Intervention is clearly stated with sufficient detail and is relevant to the problem or patient, and/or aligned to current practice.				
Comparison is clearly stated and is appropriate and relevant to the problem or patient. Comparison is gold standard of care/ or accepted usual practice/or a main alternative therapy to the proposed intervention.				
Outcome is clearly relevant to the problem or patient and is described in measurable terms that report a change, describe a rate of occurrence, adverse outcomes, or risk of occurrence. ie., decrease in blood glucose level; increase in clinical attachment level; decrease in gingival index				
Type of Question is consistently identified correctly related to levels of evidence and study methodology. Clearly understands the type of research study design that will correctly answer the PICO question.				

1. 3 new concepts I learned.

2. What is still confusing?

3. What can I do to eliminate confusion?

4. What was confusing in Chapter #_____ became clear when I...

2. The second assessment tool is **Translating Evidence Into Practice,** which allows students to document and monitor their stage of competence over a period of time. For example, beginning with skill 1, formulating a good question, students can document patient problems and the PICO questions investigated. With skill 2, a computerized search, they can document their search strategy and the evidence found. With skill 3, critical appraisal, they can record their evaluation of the evidence found and decide if it will contribute to or influence their clinical decision-making. If relevant, they can then chronical how they have applied the evidence to a patient encounter (skill4) and then evaluate the outcomes of the treatment and track their progress in using the evidence-based approach (skill 5). Ultimately, implementation of EBDM has the potential to foster translation of research findings into clinical practice, reduce variability of care provided, and improve patient health outcomes. Implementation of EBDM instruction and practice into the clinical setting has the greatest potential to achieve these improvements in patient outcomes.[1]

> ### EBDM IN PRACTICE:
>
> Evaluating the process is an important step in developing competence. It allows a practitioner an opportunity to reflect on the effectiveness of EBDM for each specific patient interaction that involves the evidence-based process.

CONCLUSION

Although the final skill in the EBDM process is evaluation of the process and your performance, it is critical to begin with a discussion of self-assessment in order to document the development of competency over time. The path for developing expertise in any skill involves learning the basic steps followed by practice in applying the skills. Reflective practitioners are continually self-assessing the results of their actions to enhance their abilities and to develop expertise. This also is the case with development of skills in EBDM. The practitioner who takes time to apply and evaluate the results of EBDM will develop expertise and foster optimal patient care.

Chapter 1 Assignments

1.   **Answer the following Critical Thinking Questions:**
        a. Why is reflection an important aspect of developing skills?
        b. How can the stages of competence guide your learning?
        c. How do portfolios help document the development of competency?

2.   **Answer the following Self-Reflection Questions:**

        a. How will I learn differently now that I understand stages of competency?
        b. What are the learning targets I have for myself in learning EBDM?
        c. What are my goals for learning this course material and what is the first step I will take to reach my goals?

        Please state your goals using S.M.A.R.T. Goal Criteria:

        S – Specific (What exactly do I want to accomplish?)
        M- Measurable (includes a number)
        A – Action (What will I do to reach my goal?)
        R – Realistic (Not too hard, but is a challenge)
        T – Timeline (When will I reach my goal?)

References

1. Booth A, Brice A. Chapter 11, "Evaluating your performance" in Evidence Based practice for information professionals: A Handbook. London: Facet Publishing, 2004. Accessed online September 18, 2015. Available at: http://www.academia.edu/225730/Evidence_Based_Practice_for_Information_Professionals_A_Handbook

2. Dreyfus Peña A. The Dreyfus model of clinical problem-solving skills acquisition: a critical perspective. Med Educ Online. 2010 Jun 14;15. doi:10.3402/meo.v15i0.4846. Review. PubMed PMID: 20563279; PubMed Central PMCID: PMC2887319.

3. American Dental Association Commission on Dental Accreditation. Accreditation Standards for Dental Education Programs, 2018. Available at http://www.ada.org/coda, Accessed 1-27-19.

4. American Dental Association Commission on Dental Accreditation. Accreditation Standards for Dental Hygiene Education Programs, 2018. Available at http://www.ada.org/coda, Accessed 1-27-19.

5. Hendricson WD, Andrieu SC, Chadwick G, et al. Educational strategies associated with development of problem-solving, critical thinking, and self-directed learning. J Dent Educ 2006; 70: 925-936.

6. Snadden D, Thomas M. The use of portfolio learning in medical education. Medical Teacher 1998;20(3):192-199.

7. Paulson FL, Paulson PP, Meyer CA. What makes a portfolio a portfolio? Educational Leadership, 1991; 48(5):60-63.

8. Dawson, Phillip (December 2015). "Assessment rubrics: towards clearer and more replicable design, research and practice Phillip". Assessment & Evaluation in Higher Education,. doi:10.1080/02602938.2015.1111294.

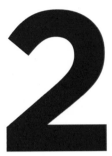

CHAPTER 2

INTRODUCTION TO EVIDENCE-BASED DECISION MAKING

Evidence-Based Decision Making Skills: Ask, Access, Appraise, Apply, Assess

Content Outline:
Purpose & Definition of EBDM
New Educational Standards
EBDM Skills & 5 Step Process
EBDM in Clinical Practice
Conclusion
Assignments
References

Learning Objectives:
Upon completion of this unit, the participant should be able to:
1. Define Evidence-based Decision Making and its purpose.
2. Identify two principles of EBDM.
3. Describe the 5 steps and skills necessary for EBDM.
4. Discuss the benefits of EBDM.

Suggested Assignments:
Online Course Dentalcare.com
Critical Thinking Questions
Self-Reflection Questions

The purpose of this chapter is to introduce basic concepts and define evidence-based decision-making [EBDM]. It provides an overview of the five steps and skills involved in establishing an evidence-based practice. Understanding the basic concepts used in EBDM builds the foundation for developing the necessary skills needed to use the process.

DDS/DMD CODA STANDARDS
EDUCATIONAL ENVIRONMENT, Critical Thinking: The components of critical thinking are: the application of logic and accepted intellectual standards to reasoning; the ability to access and evaluate evidence; the application of knowledge in clinical reasoning; and a disposition for inquiry that includes openness, self-assessment, curiosity, skepticism, and dialogue.
EDUCATIONAL ENVIRONMENT, Evidence-based Care: Evidence-based dentistry (EBD) is an approach to oral health care that requires the judicious integration of systematic assessments of clinically relevant scientific evidence, relating to the patient's oral and medical condition and history, with the dentist's clinical expertise and the patient's treatment needs and preferences.
Critical Thinking, 2-10 Graduates must be competent in the use of critical thinking and problem solving, including their use in the comprehensive care of patients, scientific inquiry and research methodology;
Clinical Sciences, 2-22- Graduates must be competent to access, critically appraise, apply and communicate scientific and lay literature as it relates to providing evidence-based patient care.
Patient Care Services, 5-2 Patient care must be evidenced-based, integrating the best research evidence and patient values.

DH CODA STANDARDS
Critical Thinking, 2-22: Graduates must be competent in the evaluation of current scientific literature.
Intent: Dental hygienists should be able to evaluate scientific literature as a basis for life-long learning, evidenced-based practice and as a foundation for adapting to changes in healthcare.
Critical Thinking, 2-23: Graduates must be competent in problem solving strategies related to comprehensive patient care and management of patients.
Intent: Critical thinking and decision-making skills are necessary to provide effective and efficient dental hygiene services.
Example: demonstration of the use of active learning methods that promote critical appraisal of scientific evidence in combination with clinical application and patient factors.

PURPOSE AND DEFINITION OF EBDM

As evidence-based medicine (EBM) has evolved, so has the realization that the evidence from scientific research is only one key component of the decision-making process and does not tell a practitioner what to do.   The use of current best evidence does not replace clinical expertise or input from the patient, but rather provides another dimension to the decision-making process that is also placed in context with the patient's clinical circumstances, Figure 2-1.

It is this decision-making process that is termed **Evidence-Based Decision Making (EBDM)** and is defined as the formalized process of using the skills for identifying, searching for and interpreting the results of the best scientific evidence, which is considered in conjunction with the clinician's experience and judgment, the patient's preferences and values, and the clinical/patient circumstances when making patient care decisions.[3] EBDM is not unique to medicine or any specific health discipline, but represents a concise way of referring to the application of evidence to the decision-making process.

Evidence-based decision-making (EBDM) is about solving clinical problems and involves two fundamental principles:[4]
1. Evidence alone is never sufficient to make a clinical decision, and
2. A hierarchy of evidence exists to guide clinical decision-making.

EBDM recognizes that clinicians can never have complete knowledge about all conditions, medications, materials or available products and provides a mechanism for assimilating current research findings into everyday practice in order to provide the best possible patient care.

NEW EDUCATIONAL STANDARDS

The ADA CODA Accreditation Standards for both Dental and Dental Hygiene Education Programs expect programs to develop specific competencies that are reflective of the evidence-based process in making patient care decisions. The evidence based (EB) process is incorporated into several areas of the Predoctoral standards, beginning with the description of the Goals of the Standards, Educational Environment and the core principles in such areas as Critical Thinking, Self-Directed Learning, Scientific Discovery and Integration of Knowledge, and Evidence-based Care.[1] For Dental Hygiene programs, the evidence-based process is incorporated into the Patient Care Competencies in order to provide patient-centered treatment that minimizes risks and optimizes oral health (Standard 2-13).[2]

Core competencies, identified by both the ADA CODA and the American Dental Education Association (ADEA) for entry-level practitioners, focus on the need for graduates to become critical thinkers, problem solvers, and consumers of current research findings to the point that they become lifelong learners. These skills parallel those of evidence-based practice by teaching

Figure 2-1 EBDM Process

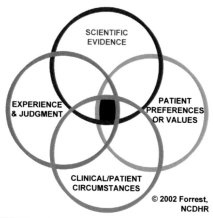

© 2002 Forrest, NCDHR

highest quality of clinically relevant research

ability to use clinical skills and past experience to rapidly identify each patient's unique health state and diagnosis, individual risks and benefits of potential interventions, personal values and expectations.

an individual's clinical condition including disease severity and prognosis that must be considered when developing treatment plan options.

unique preferences, concerns and expectations that each patient brings to a clinical encounter, including culture, language, religion, etc.

students to find, evaluate and incorporate current evidence into their decision-making. This module series builds upon the core competencies in its approach to learning and using EBDM.

EBDM SKILLS AND THE 5-STEP PROCESS

EBDM is based on the abilities to critically appraise and correctly apply current evidence from relevant research to decisions made in practice so that what is known is reflected in the care provided. It includes the process of systematically finding, appraising, and using current research findings in making clinical decisions. This requires understanding new concepts and developing new skills, such as asking good clinical questions, conducting an efficient computerized search, critically appraising the evidence, applying the results in clinical practice, and evaluating the outcomes.[5] (Table 2-1).

SKILLS NEEDED TO APPLY THE EBDM PROCESS

1. ASK: Converting information needs/problems into clinical questions so that they can be answered

The evidence-based approach guides clinicians in structuring well-built questions that result in patient-centered answers that can improve the quality of care and patient satisfaction. Asking the right question is a difficult skill to learn, yet it is fundamental to evidence-based practice. The process almost always begins with a patient question or problem. A "well-built" question should include four parts, referred to as PICO that identify the patient problem or population (P), intervention (I), comparison (C) and outcome(s) (O). This step in the process is critical to an efficient search of the literature since it identifies the key terms and outcomes that are important to identifying research studies that answer the question.

This step also requires the practitioner to classify the clinical question. The categories of classification include: therapy, diagnosis, etiology/harm, or prognosis. For example, the research design method used to answer a therapy question is not the same as the research method used to answer a diagnosis or prognosis question. Understanding the research design methodologies is a key component of being a consumer of evidence. This will be explained more fully in sections that review research designs and where research designs are directly linked to conducting an efficient search.

2. ACCESS: Conducting a computerized search with maximum efficiency for finding the best external evidence with which to answer the question

Efficiently finding relevant evidence requires conducting a very focused search of the scientific literature. Understanding where to begin the search, such as with the PubMed Clinical Queries feature, rather than with the general PubMed search box, and the use the terminology, filters, and features of scientific databases maximizes the effectiveness of the search process. In addition to PubMed, (the largest biomedical databases), there are several other online resources that can be used to find answers clinical questions. It is often necessary to use more than one online resource to find the most appropriate and highest level of evidence. For example, the DARE (Database of Abstracts of Reviews of Effects)

Table 2-1 EBDM 5 Skills

1. **ASK:** Convert information needs/problems into clinical questions so that they can be answered

2. **ACCESS:** Conduct a computerized search with maximum efficiency for finding the best external evidence with which to answer the question

3. **APPRAISE:** Critically appraise the evidence for its validity and usefulness (clinical applicability)

4. **APPLY:** Apply the results of the appraisal, or evidence, in clinical practice

5. **ASSESS:** Evaluate the process and your performance

CLINICAL APPLICATION:

Imagine a patient refused to have x-rays because they saw on the news that it caused a certain type of brain cancer.

- How would you respond?

- How would EBDM help guide your response to this patient?

www.crd.york.ac.uk/crdweb/ houses critically appraised synopses of systematic reviews, all of which are not indexed in PubMed/MEDLINE. The DARE database is housed at the University of York in Great Britain in its Centre of Reviews and Dissemination, CRD, www.evidence.nhs.uk/.

Other databases and sources of high level evidence, including clinical practice guidelines, can be found using the Trip (Translating Research into Practice) database, www.tripdatabase.com, the ADA's Center for EBD, ebd.ada.org, and the websites of specialty organizations, such the American Academy of Periodontology (AAP), www.perio.org, and the American Academy of Pediatric Dentistry (AAPD), www.aapd.org. Chapter six will detail this process more fully.

3. APPRAISE: Critically appraising the evidence for its validity and usefulness---clinical applicability

Once you have found the most current evidence, the next step in the EBDM process is to understand what you have and its relevance to your patient and PICO question. Knowing what constitutes the highest levels of evidence and having a basic understanding of research design are the foundation of acquiring the skills to appraise the scientific literature in order to answer questions and keep current with practice. Worksheets are available to guide the critical appraisal process through prompts that aid in determining the strengths, weaknesses, and validity of a study.

In addition to understanding research methodology, it also is important to understand the difference between statistical significance and clinical significance prior to deciding whether to incorporate the evidence found into your clinical decision. These are a few of the skills that are developed through the use and incorporation of critical appraisal.

4. APPLY: Applying the results of the appraisal, or evidence, in clinical practice

A key component of the fourth step is determining whether the findings are relevant to the patient, problem or question. Presenting information to patients in a clear and unambiguous manner will help translate research into practice. Health literacy is an element that is receiving significantly more attention at this time. Exercises within this series will provide simulations to practice this step in the process. The final module will assess actual patient encounters that demonstrate the discussion of evidence-based findings with actual patients.

5. ASSESS: Evaluating the process and your performance

After making a decision and implementing a course of treatment, evaluating the outcome(s) is the final step. Evaluating the process may include a range of activities such as examining outcomes related to the health/function of the patient, patient satisfaction and participation during the decision-making process, and a self-evaluation of how well each step of the EBDM process was conducted. With an understanding of how to effectively use EBDM, one can quickly and conveniently stay current with scientific findings on topics that are important to patients and the practice.

Patients come to their appointments educated and many times misinformed about new dental products, treatment procedures and diagnostic tests that they have learned about through advertisements, Internet and television. However, many of the resources available to the general public may be biased, inaccurate, or not appropriate for the patient. It is important for practitioners to develop the skills to analyze and evaluate these sources in order to accurately address patient's concerns with valid evidence. The ability to do this while integrating good science with clinical judgment enhances credibility, builds trust and confidence with the patient, and may enhance the patient's quality of care.

EBDM IN CLINICAL PRACTICE

EBDM provides a strategy for improving the efficiency of integrating new evidence into patient care by helping manage an increasing amount of information. EBDM assists in developing and providing treatment and advice that are scientifically defensible. In addition, it helps insure that practice is continually informed and strengthened by current research findings, helping to close the gap between what is known (research evidence) and what is practiced.

EBDM is not about knowing all the answers, but rather about knowing how to structure good questions to be able to find relevant information to better inform your decision making, and how and when to integrate new thinking and action into everyday practice.

CONCLUSION

Through this approach there is an understanding of how the literature should be appraised and what constitutes good evidence. Using this foundation of EBDM helps assure that practices are clinically sound and focused on the best possible outcomes. Evidence-based practice also contributes to continuously improving the effectiveness, appropriateness and quality of care. This allows practices to be consistent with risk management principles and easily substantiate the care provided to patients, policy-makers and insurance companies.

An EBDM approach closes the gap between clinical research and the realities of practice by providing dental practitioners with the skills to find, efficiently filter, interpret and apply research findings so that what is known is reflected in the treatment provided. This approach assists clinicians in keeping current with conditions a patient may have by providing a mechanism for addressing gaps in knowledge in order to provide the best care possible. For an EBDM approach to become the norm for practice it must be integrated throughout educational programs and used in developing sound clinical guidelines. Students and practitioners must learn how to learn for a lifetime of practice so that current evidence is considered and patient outcomes are optimized.

EBDM IN PRACTICE:

A dentist in a state-of-the-art practice in Deer Park, WA is using EBDM. When questions arise from patients or staff, the dentist and hygienists incorporate current scientific evidence into their decision-making process. For example, when a hygienist questioned why floss was the only inter-proximal method being recommended when other devices might be more effective in removing plaque, they turned to the current scientific literature and then presented the findings to the entire staff at an office meeting for discussion. In another case, a patient presented with Burning Mouth Syndrome (BMS) and again, the scientific literature was used to find evidence on options to relieve the BMS symptoms. Recently, a patient with severe periodontal disease questioned if hormone replacement therapy would decrease her bone loss. Again, the EBDM process was used to answer the patient's question.

Evidence Based Decision-Making Process Algorithm

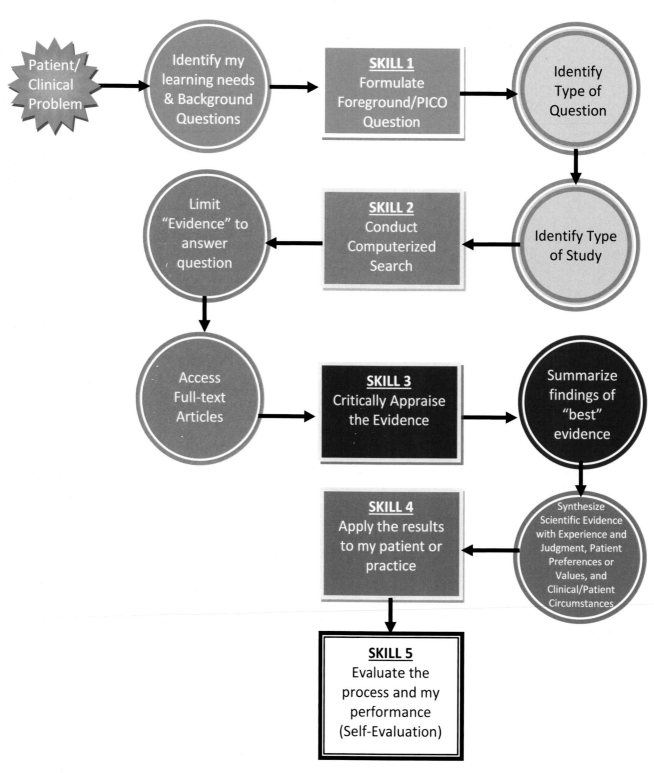

Chapter 2 Assignments

1.   **Complete the Online Tutorial:**
EBDM: Intro and Formulating Good Clinical Questions (course #311). Access via **http://www.dentalcare.com**

Focus on the overall learning objectives for this course, which are to:

a. Increase the knowledge of evidence-based concepts, principles and skills, and

b. Specifically how to formulate a good clinical question in order to find relevant evidence to answer that question.

Instructions if set up as an assignment by the course instructor:
1. Go to: **http://www.dentalcare.com**
2. Register on the site if you already have not done so. The only email you will get from the site is notification when new courses have been added. You must be registered to take the Quiz at the end of the course and receive a Certificate.
3. Under **Professional Education**, click on **Take a Course**.
4. Scroll down the page to where it says **Students Only** and **enter the assignment number** and click **GO**.
5. Once on the course site, click on **TAKE COURSE NOW**
6. There also is the option to Download the course (pdf) to save for future reference and study.
7. **Upon successful completion of the Quiz, you will be emailed a certificate. Save it for verification.** (OPTION: Print it out and bring to class or email to instructor.)

General Instructions without an Assignment Number:
1. Go to: **http://www.dentalcare.com**
2. Register on the site if you already have not done so. The only email you will get from the site is notification when new courses have been added. You must be registered to take the Quiz at the end of the course and receive a Certificate.
3. Under **Professional Education**, click on **Take a Course**.
4. Under **FIND THE RIGHT COURSE FOR YOU** there are 4 options: Select Topic, Select Audience Type, Select Author, Select Title. In this case, click on **Select Author** and scroll down to **Forrest, Jane L.** and click on **GO**.
5. Three courses are listed, so select the course you need to complete, e.g., **Evidence-based Decision Making: Introduction and Formulating Good Clinical Questions**
6. Click on **Take a Course**
7. There also is the option to Download the course (pdf) to save for future reference and study.
8. **Upon successful completion of the Quiz, you will be emailed a Certificate. Save it for verification. (OPTION: Print it out and bring to class or email to instructor.)**

Chapter 2 Assignments

2.   **Answer the following Critical Thinking Questions:**

    a.   Describe a situation when the EBDM process is helpful in finding answers for a question.

    b.   Discuss how EBDM influences dental and dental hygiene practice today.

    c.   Identify and discuss 3 primary reasons EBDM is critical for health care providers.

3.   **Answer the following Self-Reflection Questions:**

    a.   What was the one most useful thing you learned in this chapter?

    b.   How does the EBDM process improve your ability as a critical thinker?

    c.   How is learning about EBDM beneficial to you?

References

1. American Dental Association Commission on Dental Acreditation. Accreditation Standards for Dental Education Programs (Predoctoral). Chicago: ADA, 2010. Accessed 9-5-15, **www.ada.org/en/coda/current-accreditation-standards**

2. American Dental Association Commission on Dental Accreditation. Accreditation Standards for Allied Dental Education Programs (Dental Hygiene). Chicago: ADA, 2013. Accessed 9-5-15, **www.ada.org/en/coda/current-accreditation-standards**

3. Forrest JL, Miller SA, Overman PR, Newman MG. Evidence-Based Decision-Making: A Translational Guide for Dental Professionals.   Philadelphia: Lippincott Williams & Wilkins, 2009.

4. Guyatt G, Drummond R, Meade M, Cook D. Evidence-based Medicine Working Group. Users' Guides to the Medical Literature, A Manual for Evidence-Based Clinical Practice. 2nd ed. (JAMA & Archives Journals), Chicago: McGraw Hill Medical, 2008.

5. Straus S, Richardson W, Glasziou P, Haynes RB. Evidence-Based Medicine: How to Practice and Teach EBM. 4th ed. London, England: Churchill Livingstone, 2010.

NOTES

CHAPTER

3

THE PICO PROCESS

Skill 1. ASK: Converting Information Needs Problems into Clinical Questions so that they can be answered

Content Outline:
Background and Foreground Questions
Four Parts of a PICO Question
Four types of Questions
Conclusion
Assignments
References

Learning Objectives:
Upon completion of this chapter, the reader should be able to:
1. Identify characteristics of Background and Foreground Questions.
2. Given example questions, accurately identify it as a Background or Foreground question.
3. Given example questions, accurately identify each component of a PICO question.
4. Identify characteristics of four types of PICO questions- therapy, harm, prognosis, diagnosis.

Suggested Assignments:
PICO & Type of Question Wksht
Critical Thinking Questions
Self-Reflection Questions

The purpose of this chapter is to discuss PICO, a systematic process for converting information needs or problems into clinical questions so that they can be answered. This is a fundamental step in the EBDM because it forces the questioner to focus on the most important single issue and outcome, and it facilitates the identification of key search terms.

DDS/DMD CODA STANDARDS
EDUCATIONAL ENVIRONMENT, Critical Thinking: Identify problems & formulate questions clearly and precisely.

EDUCATIONAL ENVIRONMENT, Evidence-based Care: Evidence-based dentistry (EBD) is an approach to oral health care that requires the judicious integration of systematic assessments of clinically relevant scientific evidence, relating to the patient's oral and medical condition and history, with the dentist's clinical expertise and the patient's treatment needs and preferences.

Critical Thinking, 2-10 Graduates must be competent in the use of critical thinking and problem solving, including their use in the comprehensive care of patients, scientific inquiry and research methodology;

Patient Care Services, 5-2 Patient care must be evidenced-based, integrating the best research evidence and patient values.

DH CODA STANDARDS
Critical Thinking, 2-23: Graduates must be competent in problem solving strategies related to comprehensive patient care and management of patients.

BACKGROUND AND FOREGROUND QUESTIONS

Background questions are general knowledge inquiries that ask who, what, where, when, how, or why. They are used to help narrow a broad scope and search about a topic in order to find the details needed for a foreground/specific (PICO) question. A background question may be necessary to identify specific interventions for a disease or problem or to learn more about one particular disorder, intervention or drug therapy. These questions are helpful in identifying articles that provide more specific details that can be used in developing foreground questions. Finding a good article that reviews the management of a problem often provides the necessary details. Often these can be quickly answered using a general Internet search engine.

Examples of background questions include:
- What causes _____(identify disease OR condition)?
- What is _____(identify product or therapy)?
- How are patients with_____(identify disease or condition treated/managed?
- What are suggested therapies for _____ (identify disease problem)?

A foreground question often arises from a problem or patient question. It is a specific question that is structured to find a precise answer and phrased to facilitate a computerized search. A "well-built" or foreground question should include four parts that identify the

1. Patient and/or problem (P),
2. Intervention (I),
3. Comparison (C) [a 2nd intervention, typically the gold standard for treatment or diagnosis], and
4. Outcome(s) (O).

This question is referred to as PICO[1] and is often generated directly by the patient or the treatment being considered. However, it also can emerge from an observed problem, a topic of interest, or to explore a new material or procedure, to clarify differences, or compare cost-effectiveness.[2] Foreground or PICO questions are the first step in finding valid scientific evidence to answer a clinical question. The differences between background and foreground questions are contrasted in Table 3-1.

APPLICATION OF QUESTIONS

EXAMPLE CASE: Nathan, a 73-year-old male patient is complaining of a burning sensation on his lips and tongue. He is diagnosed to have burning mouth syndrome. This is the clinician's first encounter with burning mouth syndrome. The patient wants to know if the clinician can help relieve the burning.

Sample Background Questions:
1. What is burning mouth syndrome?
2. What causes burning mouth syndrome?
3. What is the recommended treatment for burning mouth syndrome?

Table 3-1 Differences between Background & Foreground Questions

BACKGROUND VS. FOREGROUND	
General knowledge, broad	Specific
Asks who, what, where, when, how, or why	Identifies each P, I, C, O component
Helps to narrow a broad scope	Structured to find a precise answer and phrased to facilitate a computerized search
Used to find articles that provide more specific details to a broad question	Identifies valid evidence to answer a specific question

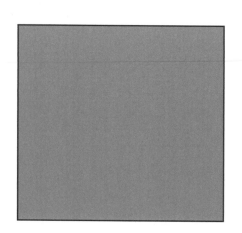

A basic search engine or smartphone "intelligent assistant" can help find answers to these sample background questions. If you need additional help, online answers can be found on the American Family Physician website at **http://www.aafp.org**

FOUR PARTS OF A PICO QUESTION

The PICO process was developed to convert information needs or problems into specific clinical questions so that they can be answered, the first step in the evidence-based (EB) approach.

Asking the right question is perhaps the hardest skill to learn, and yet it is fundamental to the evidence-based decision-making process. As previously mentioned, the formality of using PICO to frame the question serves three key purposes because it:

1. Compels the clinician to focus on what the patient/client believes to be the most important single issue and outcome.
2. Facilitates the 2nd step in the EB process, the computerized search, by identifying key terms that will be used in the search.[1]
3. Requires a clear identification of the problem, results and outcomes related to the specific care being considered for that patient. This, in turn, helps to determine the type of evidence and information required to solve the problem and to measure the effectiveness of the intervention.

One of the greatest difficulties in developing each aspect of the PICO question is providing an adequate amount of information without being too detailed. It is important to stay focused on the main components that directly affect the situation. Each component of a PICO question should be specific, but not merely a laundry list of everything regarding that problem or patient. Each component of the PICO question should be stated as a specific term or a concise short phrase.

PROBLEM/PATIENT POPULATION

The first step in developing a well-built question is to identify the patient problem or patient population, which typically is either the **patient's chief complaint or disease/condition that requires treatment or prevention.** It is helpful to consider the following when identifying the P in PICO.

1. How you would describe the patient/problem/condition to a colleague?
2. What are the most important characteristics of this patient/ problem?
3. Primary Problem
4. Patient's main concern or chief complaint
5. Disease/condition (including severity) or health status
6. Age, Race, Gender, Previous ailments, current medications
7. Which of these characteristics should be considered as I search for evidence? [1]

PICO Components for Nathan

P **burning mouth syndrome**

Age and gender may be included but are not essential details.

For some questions it also may be appropriate to identify a general population instead of focusing on a patient or chief complaint. Population refers to the characteristics of the patient that differentiate them from the general public. For example, specific question may investigate pregnant women or non-fluoridated communities. It describes the specific attributes a researcher would be looking for when conducting a research study.

The **P** component could be more detailed if the components influence the results of the search. These may include the characteristics of age, gender, health history or medications. For example, it may be necessary to clarify the patient as an adult in the case of periodontitis or a middle-aged female if the results are regarding postmenopausal women. However, it is usually easier to keep each component as basic as possible so as not to exclude relevant citations when searching the literature. Specific characteristics of the **P** component are helpful when appraising the literature and then applying the findings to patients to verify that the studies are applicable and appropriate.

INTERVENTION

Identifying the Intervention is the second step in the PICO process. It is important to identify **what new/main treatment option is being considered or what the patient is asking about,** which keeps the process patient-centered. This may include the use of a new specific diagnostic test, treatment, adjunctive therapy, medication or the recommendation to the patient to use a product or procedure. The Intervention is the **new/main consideration** for that patient or client.[1]

COMPARISON

The third component of a well-built question is the Comparison, which is the second treatment/intervention option being considered.[1] The Comparison should be specific and limited to **one alternative choice** in order to facilitate an effective computerized search. One may only look at the Intervention without exploring alternatives to learn more about it; however, when there is a comparison it should be used. The Comparison is treatment typically provided, which hopefully is the gold standard or standard of care. When more than one option is available, it is important to select only the most appropriate **one**. Avoid multiple topics in one clinical question

OUTCOME

The final component is the Outcome. This specifies the result(s) of what you plan to accomplish, improve or affect. In other words, it should **solve the problem**. Outcomes should be **measurable** and may consist of relieving or eliminating specific symptoms, improving or maintaining function, enhancing esthetics and/or preventing disease. **Specific** outcomes also will yield better search results. When defining the outcome, *more effective* is not acceptable unless it describes *how* the intervention is effective, e.g., more effective in decreasing caries incidence, or more effective in preventing tooth fractures. The outcome should relate directly to the patient or problem.

PICO Components for Nathan

I tricyclic antidepressants

Multiple options were found from the background search however only **ONE** intervention should be selected

C benzodiazepines

Specific medications within the drug class can be selected- but may limit the results in a search.

O more effective in **relieving the burning sensation on his lips and tongue**

FORMULA FOR WRITING PICO QUESTIONS

There is a "specific formula" for writing a PICO question. Most can be written using the following structure and filling in the blanks with the P-I-C-O components previously identified:

For a patient with specific problem/population **(P), will** what you plan to do **(I), compared to** main alternative/gold standard **(C) result in** measurable results that solve the P problem **(O)?**

FOUR TYPES OF QUESTIONS

Clinical evidence is primarily derived from questions that address therapy/prevention, diagnosis, harm (also known as etiology or causation), and prognosis. Identifying the type of question facilitates understanding the type of research studies that will best answer the question and how to filter the search to find studies more efficiently.

Therapy/Prevention questions look for answers that determine the effect of treatments/interventions that are important outcomes for patients, e.g., improve function, are worth the effort and cost, and that prevent harm or avoid adverse events.

Example:
For a patient with oral squamous cell carcinoma and periodontal disease in the posterior region, will extraction of the periodontally involved molars, as compared to periodontal treatment, be more effective in promoting long-term stability?

Diagnosis questions look for evidence to determine the degree to which a test is reliable and useful. The selection and interpretation of diagnostic methods or tests that establish the power of an intervention to differentiate between those with and without the condition or disease is the aim of diagnosis questions.

Example:
For a patient with a suspicious oral lesion, will use of a Velscope (fluorescence imaging) as compared to visual screening and palpation be more effective in earlier detection of a cancerous lesion?

Harm, Etiology, Causation questions are used to identify causes of a disease or condition including iatrogenic forms and to determine relationships between risk factors, potentially harm-ful agents, and possible causes of a disease or condition.

Example:
For a patient with oral cancer undergoing head and neck radia-tion, will fluoride treatments prior to and after radiation treat-ment, as compared to fluoride treatments only after radiation treatment, be more effective in reducing the risk of dry mouth and caries?

PICO Question for Nathan

> For a patient with **burning mouth syndrome**, will **tricyclic anti-depressants,** compared to **benzodiazepines**, be more effective in **relieving the burning sensation on his lips and tongue**?

PRACTICE SKILLS:

Write an alternative PICO question for Nathan. Use a different Intervention and Comparison based on the specific findings from the background question.

For a patient with burning mouth syndrome, will (new I)

_____

compared to (new C)

_____

be more effective in relieving the burning sensation on his lips and tongue?

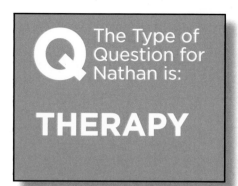

The Type of Question for Nathan is:

THERAPY

Prognosis questions look to studies that estimate the clinical course or progression of a disease or condition over time and anticipate likely complications (and prevent them).

Example:
Is a patient who has been treated for oral cancer, as compared to someone who has not had oral cancer, at greater risk of losing teeth?

In questions of prognosis, the Intervention is typically the risk factor, such as those with a prior oral cancer. The Comparison is the absence of this risk factor, i.e., those without a prior oral cancer.

An educational tool will be used throughout this module series to guide the learner through the steps of evidence-based decision-making. An example of the first portion of this tool is found in Figure 3-1. This will tool be used throughout the following chapters to guide learning and reinforce concepts.

CONCLUSION

PICO is a systematic process for converting information needs/problems into clinical questions that defines the patient problem, intervention, comparison and outcome. In addition to understanding how to ask a clinical question, identifying the type of question, such as therapy, diagnosis, harm or prognosis helps to know what is being asked. These steps in asking PICO questions establish a solid groundwork for finding the appropriate scientific evidence to answer the questions.

Table 3-2. Translating Evidence into Practice Tool

Name <u>Syrene Miller</u>   Topic <u>Burning Mouth Syndrome</u>

1. **Write Background question**s - general knowledge inquiries that ask who, what, where, when, how, or why that you need to learn more about.

   1. What is burning mouth syndrome (BMS)?
   2. What causes BMS?
   3. How is BMS diagnosed?
   4. What are the suggested therapies for BMS?

2. **Summarize the findings from the Background questions.**
   1. BMS is a common problem especially in women during or after menopause. People with BMS feel a bitter or metallic taste in their mouth or feel like they burned their mouth.

   2. Researchers are not sure of the cause, however they think it may be a problem in the nerves that control taste and pain.

   3. There is no simple way to diagnose BMS. The doctor may rule out a problem that may be causing a burning sensation.

   4. BMS may be treated with antidepressants like amitriptyline or benzodiazepines. Capsaicin is a hot pepper mouth rinse that may help. Other interventions investigated are alpha-lipoic acid and hormone replacement therapy.

3. **Outline the PICO question** by identifying: Problem, Intervention, Comparison and Outcome(s). This question will be used to establish a search strategy.

   Patient/Population   <u>burning mouth syndrome</u>

   Intervention   <u>tricyclic antidepressants</u>

   Comparison   <u>benzodiazepines</u>

   Outcome   <u>relieve burning sensation on lips and tongue</u>

4. **Write a PICO (foreground) question:**
   For a patient with burning mouth syndrome, will tricyclic antidepressants compared to benzodiazepines, be more effective in relieving the burning sensation on the lips and tongue?

5. **Identify the Type of question** appropriate for your patient. Circle one:

   (Therapy/Prevention)   Diagnosis   Etiology, Causation, or Harm   Prognosis

Table 3-3. Relationship of type of Question and PICO Components

Question Type	Patient, Problem	Intervention or Exposure	Comparison	Outcome Measures
Treatment (Therapy)/ Prevention	The patient's disease or condition, e.g., caries, perio, diabetes. OR The patient's risk factors (smoker, nutrition, habits) and general health condition.	A therapeutic or preventive measure medication, material, restorative or surgical tmt, or a behavioral change.	Gold standard of care, or accepted standard of practice, or a placebo.	Reduction or improvement in the disease or condition. E.g., morbidity rate, days lost from work/school, tooth loss, pain, functionality, disease incidence.
Diagnosis	The target or suspected disease or condition, e.g., oral cancer	A new diagnostic test or procedure.	The current "gold standard" test for the problem, biopsy.	Measures the new Dx test in comparison with the "gold standard."
Prognosis (Natural History)	The main clinical problem in terms of its severity and duration, e.g., bone loss, prior history of oral cancer.	The exposure of interest is usually the risk factor and time.	A comparable intervention; may not be applicable.	Ex: survival rates, mortality or morbidity rates, rates disease progression, e.g., bone loss or development of a new cancer.
Etiology or Harm (Causation)	Your patient's risk factors, e.g., overhanging restoration; current health disorder, e.g., gingivitis, or general health condition.	The intervention or exposure of interest, including some indication of dose strength of the risk factor duration of the exposure, or type of material.	A comparable intervention; may not be applicable.	Ex: disease incidence, rates of disease progression, morbidity rates.

Adapted from Guyatt G, Meade MO, Richardson S, Jaeschke R. Chapter 3. What is the question? In: Guyatt G, Rennie D, Meade MO, Cook DJ, eds. Users' Guides to the Medical Literature: A Manual for Evidence-Based Clinical Practice. 2nd ed. New York, NY: McGraw-Hill; 2008.

Chapter 3 Assignments - The PICO Process

1. **Complete the Exercise 1 - PICO & Type of Question**

2. Briefly write about a situation, topic, or patient/ problem for which you do not have answers or need more complete information. Second, write what you consider to be the Problem, Intervention, Comparison, and Outcome. Finally, write out the PICO question to accompany the scenario.

    a. Identify a situation, topic, patient problem:

    b. Write out what you consider to be the:

          Problem:

          Intervention:

          Comparison:

          Outcome:

    c. Write out the PICO question using the specific formula:

    d. Discuss how foreground questions are useful in finding answers to clinical questions.

3. **Answer the following Self-Reflection Questions:**

    a. Am I able to generate a background question?

    b. Am I able to identify each component of a PICO or focused clinical question: Patient/Problem, Intervention, Comparison, Outcome?

    c. Am I able to differentiate the four types of clinical questions: Therapy/Prevention, Diagnosis, Prognosis, Etiology, Causation, Harm?

    d. What problems did I encounter in this chapter?

    e. What still needs further clarification?

Exercise 1 - PICO and Type of Question

Read the following PICO questions. Circle the P, underline the I, double underline the C, and highlight the outcome. Then identify the Type of Question being asked.

---

1. For adult patients with recurrent aphthous ulcers (cold sores), will a daily zinc supplement compared to a 0.12% chlorhexidine daily rinse more effectively reduce the frequency of outbursts?

Type of Question: ☐ Therapy/ Prevention ☐ Diagnosis ☐ Etiology, Causation, Harm ☐ Prognosis

---

2. For adults with dental implants, will diabetes significantly decrease the longevity of the implants?

Type of Question: ☐ Therapy/ Prevention ☐ Diagnosis ☐ Etiology, Causation, Harm ☐ Prognosis

---

3. For patients with dental caries on mandibular molars, will the placement of CEREC inlays compared to large composite restorations increase the longevity of the restoration?

Type of Question: ☐ Therapy/ Prevention ☐ Diagnosis ☐ Etiology, Causation, Harm ☐ Prognosis

---

4. For patients with malodor, will tongue brushing compared to mouth rinsing reduce the bacteria causing the malodor?

Type of Question: ☐ Therapy/ Prevention ☐ Diagnosis ☐ Etiology, Causation, Harm ☐ Prognosis

---

5. For patients with prosthetic joints, should prophylactic antibiotic coverage be prescribed prior to undergoing dental procedures to prevent infection?

Type of Question: ☐ Therapy/ Prevention ☐ Diagnosis ☐ Etiology, Causation, Harm ☐ Prognosis

---

6. For a patient with periapical bone lesions, will cone beam computed tomography (CBCT) compared to traditional intraoral radiographs, be more accurate in assessing apical bone destruction?

Type of Question: ☐ Therapy/ Prevention ☐ Diagnosis ☐ Etiology, Causation, Harm ☐ Prognosis

---

7. For managing a patient with periodontal disease, will use of a Nd:Yag compared to scaling and root planning be as effective in managing periodontal disease?

Type of Question: ☐ Therapy/ Prevention ☐ Diagnosis ☐ Etiology, Causation, Harm ☐ Prognosis

---

8. For smokers undergoing periodontal flap surgery, will the clinical healing (gain in CAL, decrease in PD) be compromised if they continue to smoke?

Type of Question: ☐ Therapy/ Prevention ☐ Diagnosis ☐ Etiology, Causation, Harm ☐ Prognosis

---

9. For a patient with dental caries will fiber-optic transillumination as compared to radiographs be more accurate in assessing dental caries?

Type of Question: ☐ Therapy/ Prevention ☐ Diagnosis ☐ Etiology, Causation, Harm ☐ Prognosis

---

10. For young children using a bottle, will a bottle with juice compared to a bottle with water increase the number of early childhood caries?

Type of Question: ☐ Therapy/ Prevention ☐ Diagnosis ☐ Etiology, Causation, Harm ☐ Prognosis

References

1. Straus SE, Glasziou P, Richardson WS, Haynes RB. Evidence-based Medicine: How to Practice and Teach it. 5th Ed. London, England: Churchill Livingstone Elsevier, 2019.

2. Richards D. Asking the right question right. Evidence-Based Dentistry 2000;2:20-21.

NOTES

CHAPTER

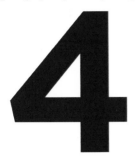

UNDERSTANDING LEVELS OF EVIDENCE:
PRIMARY RESEARCH DESIGN

Learning Objectives:
Upon completion of this chapter readers will be able to
1. Explain the difference between experimental and non-experimental research
2. Identify distinguishing characteristics of different primary research designs
3. Understand the relationship of primary research designs and their corresponding levels of evidence
4. Distinguish the difference between quantitative and qualitative research
5. Explain how each level of evidence contributes to a continuum of knowledge

Suggested Assignments:
Online Tutorials/Video
Study Design Exercise
Critical Thinking Questions
Self-Reflection Questions

Understanding research design is the foundation for using evidence in practice. It is critical to the evidence-based process in that it helps you know what you are looking for, determine the validity of the research, and decide if that evidence can be applied to the patient. The purpose of this chapter is to discuss characteristics of primary research and corresponding levels of evidence. Although EBDM emphasizes using randomized controlled trials and other quantitative methods, a brief overview of qualitative research also is presented. Secondary sources of evidence and their characteristics will be reviewed in Chapter 5.

DDS/DMD CODA STANDARDS
EDUCATIONAL ENVIRONMENT, Scientific Discovery and the Integration of Knowledge: the capacity to think scientifically and to apply the scientific method is critical if students are to analyze and solve oral health problems, understand research, and practice evidence-based dentistry.
Critical Thinking, 2-10 Graduates must be competent in the use of critical thinking and problem-solving, including their use in the comprehensive care of patients, scientific inquiry and *research methodology.*
Clinical Sciences, 2-22 Graduates must be competent to access, critically appraise, apply, and communicate scientific and lay literature as it relates to providing evidence-based patient care. Intent: The education program should introduce students to the basic principles of clinical and translational research, including how such research is conducted, evaluated, applied, and explained to patients.

DH CODA STANDARDS
Critical Thinking, 2-22: Graduates must be competent in the evaluation of current scientific literature.
Critical Thinking, 2-23: Graduates must be competent in problem solving strategies related to comprehensive patient care and management of patients.

NOT ALL EVIDENCE IS EQUAL

Levels of evidence exist in that there is a hierarchy of evidence available to guide clinical decision-making, and as a hierarchy implies, not all evidence is equally useful for making patient care decisions.

As you progress up the hierarchy, the research designs allow more control so that intervention or treatment outcome differences are not due to chance. Also, as you progress up the hierarchy, the number of published studies decreases, and yet these are more clinically relevant studies.

In Figure 4-1, the hierarchy of evidence is shown. There are two categories of evidence sources: Primary and Secondary research studies. Understanding the distinction between these two will help in searching for evidence and critically analyzing it (the third step in the EB process). This chapter will focus specifically on primary research sources, which include original individual research studies.

Figure 4-1   Hierarchy of Research Designs and Levels of Scientific Evidence

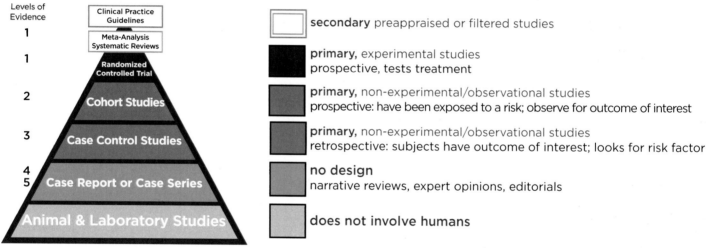

© 2016 Forrest & Miller, EBDM in Action: Developing Competence in EB Practice

The highest level of primary research is an individual RCT (Level 1). This level of evidence is followed respectively by Cohort studies (Level 2), and Case-control studies (Level 3). Case reports, narrative reviews and editorials (Levels 4 and 5) do not involve a research design. Although animal and laboratory research studies are extremely important, they are at the bottom of the hierarchy because they do not involve human subjects and evidence-based practice is all about how it works in people.

EXPERIMENTAL (OR INTERVENTIONAL) STUDIES

Beginning with the highest level of primary research, these studies involve participants that undergo an intervention in order to evaluate its impact. These experimental studies are the most methodologically challenging and ones in which the researcher controls or manipulates the variables (i.e., the intervention, its timing and dose) under investigation, such as in testing the effectiveness of a treatment, as compared to another treatment or a placebo. These studies are the most complex and include

randomized and non-randomized controlled trials. The Randomized Controlled Trial (RCT) provides the strongest evidence for **demonstrating cause and effect**, i.e., the treatment has caused the effect, rather than it happening by chance.

An RCT study design involves
- At least one test/experimental treatment or intervention, and one control treatment, which can be a placebo treatment or no treatment
- Concurrent enrollment of subjects and follow-up of the experimental and control groups
- Assignment of subjects to either the experimental treatment or intervention group or the control/placebo group through a random process, such as the use of a random-numbers table
- Follow-up of both groups to determine the outcome

The most important characteristics of RCTs are the ability to **randomly assign subjects**, i.e., each subject has an equal chance of being assigned to either the experimental or control group, and to **randomly allocate treatments**. Therefore, the groups are alike in all important aspects and the differences observed can be attributed to the treatment. Other unique features of RCTs that reduce bias and strengthen validity are that they are **prospective** (going forward in time) in nature and can include blind or double blind strategies. A **double blind RCT** is one in which neither subject nor investigator knows whether the patient is receiving the experimental treatment or the control treatment. Studies involving therapies (pills/liquids/pastes) are easy to double blind because the subject takes one of two treatments of identical size, dose, shape, and color, and neither the patient, the investigator or the assessor/examiner knows who is taking the treatment or the placebo.

Double blinding masks the allocation assignment and helps to **minimize allocation bias**, thus balancing out known and unknown variables. It also reduces the expectations of what will be observed and reported so that the results are not biased. It is more difficult to double blind studies when testing a new treatment, technique or procedure where the investigator or patient can distinguish a difference. In these studies, an examiner who has not been involved in the implementation of the study should be used to evaluate the results to decrease bias.

Non-randomized controlled trials should be used in **diagnostic studies** where the outcomes from a new test under evaluation are compared with outcomes from the reference or gold standard test, i.e., the test or measure considered the ultimate or ideal. In controlled trials there is no randomization since **both tests are given to each subject** who is suspected of having the condition of interest, and measurements from each test are compared to determine if the new test is as accurate as the reference or gold standard test. For example, comparing two different radiographic techniques/procedures, tradition film vs. digital, or digital vs. CBCT. In order to make the comparison, both techniques or procedures have to be used on the same person, in the same area of the mouth.

> **Random Assignment:**
> Each subject has an equal chance of being assigned to either the experimental or control group

NON-EXPERIMENTAL/OBSERVATIONAL STUDIES

Non-experimental or observational studies are those in which the researcher does not give a treatment, intervention or provide an exposure, i.e., data is gathered without intervening to control variables. Examples of non-experimental studies include **cohort** and **case control studies**. Case series and case reports have no control group or design, so that they are **just reports** of what has occurred.

Cohort studies make observations about the association between a particular **exposure or a risk factor** (e.g., tobacco use) and the **subsequent development of a disease or condition** (e.g., lung cancer). In these studies, subjects are selected on the basis of differences in their exposure, e.g., exposure to tobacco, smokers, or no exposure, non-smokers. **Neither group presently has the condition of interest** (lung cancer) and is followed over time to see at what frequency each develops the disease/condition under investigation (Figure 4-2).

As in experimental studies, both groups are followed prospectively and there is the ability to establish a temporal sequence for the relationship between exposure to risk factors and development of a particular disease or condition.[1]

The temporal sequence (i.e., the exposure has to precede the development of the disease/condition) is necessary for drawing inferences about causative factors. The important advantage of this design is the ability to control and monitor data collection and to measure variables accurately.

A **cohort study** is most useful where the **disease/condition of interest occurs frequently** and **subjects can be readily obtained**. It also is useful when the risk factors are known or thought to cause harm (tobacco use) and when there are **ethical considerations.** For example, researchers could not conduct an experimental study to determine if tobacco use causes lung cancer. This would require that subjects (all non-users of tobacco) be randomly assigned to an experimental or control group and those in the experimental given "x" number packs of cigarettes to smoke each day. Instead, investigators find people who **already** smoke "x" number packs of cigarettes per day (and who do not have lung cancer) and match them with as similar a group as possible, with the exception of not smoking, to serve as the control group. Both groups then are followed over time and the incidence of lung cancer in the experimental group (those who smoke) is compared with the incidence of lung cancer in the control group (those who do not smoke). Obvious disadvantages are the time that it could take to develop the disease or condition of interest (lung cancer), the cost of follow-up and the potential for losing subjects over time, which can affect the sample size and the outcomes of the statistical analysis.

Cohort studies also may be used to determine the **prognosis** of a disease/condition. However, in this situation, patients have been diagnosed with an early stage of a disease or have been successfully treated for a disease and want to know the likelihood of what will happen over time. This group is considered an

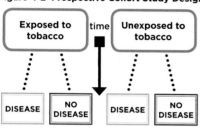

Figure 4-2 Prospective Cohort Study Design

Persons with and without the exposure of interest (e.g., tobacco) are identified at the initiation of the study. Information is then collected looking forward in time to identify outcomes, i.e. disease (lung cancer) or no disease. At the start of the study, neither group has the disease or condition of interest.

inception cohort and is followed up at certain intervals to see what has happened. For example, for those patients who have been treated for cancer, what is the incidence of developing a second cancer? Or, for those patients with diabetes, what is the likelihood of losing a tooth?

Case control studies make observations about possible associations between the disease of interest (lung cancer) and one or more hypothesized risk factors (tobacco use). Case control studies investigate subjects who **already have a certain disease or condition** and are compared with a representative group of disease-free persons (controls) from the same population.   A case control study is most **useful in studying the etiology of rare diseases** since they are difficult to study on a population basis. Also, a case study allows multiple etiologic factors to be studied concurrently.

The problem with case control studies is that they are **retrospective** (looking back in time). In these cases, investigators often have to **rely on the subjects' recall or other incomplete sources of information for exposure histories** or characteristics that could have put a person at risk for developing the condition or disease of interest. As a result, this study design lends itself to **recall bias** and extraneous variables more so than a cohort or experimental study. The assumption is that the differences should explain why the cases developed the condition/disease of interest and the controls did not. Although simplified, using the tobacco and lung cancer example, lung cancer patients would be asked questions related to their smoking history. For example, do they currently smoke, or have they every smoked and if so, when did they started smoking, how much did they and currently smoke, when did it increase and by how much, did they ever stop and then start again and when, and their answers would be compared with those of the control group.

Another example of a case control study is the one that examined the relationship between the receipt or frequency of dental radiographs and intracranial meningioma.[2] Participants were interviewed by telephone and asked to recall the number of times they received radiographs during 4 periods: younger than 10 years old, between the ages of 10-19, 20-29, and older than 50. With the average age of participants being 57, one has to question how accurate the reporting was since the information provided could not be verified. Also, a review of the methodological procedures, data analysis, and accounting for other possible explanations is incomplete.

Case control studies also are less reliable because a statistical relationship between two conditions does not mean that one condition actually caused the other. For instance, lung cancer rates may be higher for people who earn less than $50,000 per year, but that doesn't mean that someone can reduce his or her cancer risk just by getting a salary increase to over $50,000. When possible, researchers should confirm the results with a randomized controlled trial or a prospective cohort study.

Figure 4-3 Retrospective Case Control Study Design

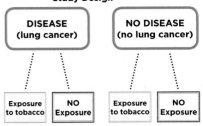

Persons **with and without the disease** of interest (e.g., lung cancer) are identified at the initiation of the study. Information is then collected looking backward in time to identify potential exposures or risk factors (e.g., tobacco) that could have contributed to getting the disease.

REAL-LIFE RESEARCH

In April 2014 Flint, Michigan, USA changed the source of their drinking water from treated water sourced from Lake Huron & the Detroit River to water sourced from the Flint River. It was reported that the new water source corroded the lead pipes and contaminated the drinking water leading to higher blood lead levels in children particulary in socio-disadvantaged neighborhoods.

1. How did initial observations in Flint, initiate structured research studies?

2. Why is a case-controlled study appropriate to investigate changes in blood lead levels?

3. How can case-control study findings generate additional research studies?

4. What **new** study design(s) should originate from these findings?

ajph.aphapublications.org/doi/abs/10.2105/AJPH.2015.303003

CASE REPORT AND CASE SERIES

Case reports and case series are often reported in the dental and dental hygiene literature. These consist either of a report of a single patient or reports on the treatment of several patients. For example if a patient has a condition that a clinician has never seen or heard of before and is uncertain what to do, a search for a case report or case series may reveal information that will assist in a diagnosis or course of treatment. However, for any reasonably well-known condition there should be better evidence.

Case reports and case series have **no research design or statistical validity, since they report observations and do not use a control group with which to compare outcomes**. However, they can be extremely important in identifying new health concerns and often generate a hypothesis that then sparks the initiation of more rigorous prospective studies and clinical trials as they did with the discovery of water fluoridation,[3] toxic shock syndrome[4] and AIDS.[5]

A summary of primary research study designs, their benefits, disadvantages and bias is illustrated in Table 4-1.

QUANTITATIVE AND QUALITATIVE RESEARCH

Primary research consists of both **quantitative** and **qualitative** research, although qualitative research is not represented in this hierarchy. Most of the research and literature related to EBDM refers to **quantitative research**, which focuses on establishing cause and effect relationships through testing a specific hypothesis and reporting the results in statistical terms. Quantitative research can be experimental or non-experimental/observational. In these types of studies the researcher tends to remain separate from the subject matter and **data are reported in numerical and statistical terms.**

In comparison, **qualitative research** is exploratory and uses an interpretive, naturalistic approach that focuses on how individuals or groups view and understand their surroundings and construct meaning out of their experiences. Qualitative research **investigates the why and how** of decision-making and the researcher tends to be immersed in the subject matter and/or there is personal involvement. Three examples of qualitative paradigms/research strategies and their related criteria are found in Table 4-2.[6]

Typical methods used include observation, structured interviews, focus groups, and consensus methods. Data are typically reported using narrative terms and not displayed mathematically in tables or graphs. For example, some participants in a focus group on oral cancer prevention and early detection when asked if they had ever received an oral cancer screening reported, "They checked the inside of my cheeks and pulled out my tongue and felt my neck. They didn't tell me what they were doing."[7]
Table 4-3 summarizes the characteristics of quantitative and qualitative research approaches.

Table 4-1. Summary of Primary Research Study Designs and Reports

Study Design	Objectives	Methods	Benefits	Disadvantages	Common Bias
Experimental Randomized Controlled Trial (Prospective)	Test interventions demonstrating cause and effect; Standard for evaluating therapeutic efficacy.	Experimental group & Control group; Randomization of subjects and treatments; blinding of subjects and investigators.	Provides strongest evidence for causality; Minimizes bias via randomization & blinding; internal and external validity	Cost, Time and Ethical considerations	Selection, Allocation, Attrition and Reporting bias
Experimental Controlled Trial (Prospective)	Determine if a new test is valid and reliable, i.e., the probability of getting a true test result given the patient has, or does not have, the disease/condition of interest.	Comparison of the new test to the gold standard. Both tests are given to the same person.	Ability to determine the sensitivity and specificity of the new test.	Cost and Time	
Non-Experimental Cohort Study (Prospective)	Observe association about exposure or risk factor & subsequent development of disease/condition; Determine diagnosis and etiology of disease.	Exposure group compared to Non-exposure group; Prospective–subjects do not have the disease/condition of interest; Measures made before disease development.	Ability to establish temporal sequence; ability to control and monitor data collection and measure variables accurately. Useful when disease/condition occurs frequently.	Time to develop disease or condition, cost of follow-up and losing subjects over time. Difficult to establish causation.	Loss to follow-up.
Non-Experimental Inception Cohort Study	Used to determine the prognosis of a disease or condition.	A defined, sample of patients assembled at a common (usually early) point in the course of their disease and free of the outcome of interest.	Ability to determine the incidence (new cases) and different outcomes.	Time to develop disease or condition, cost of follow-up and losing subjects over time.	Loss to follow-up.
Non-Experimental Case Control (Retrospective)	Observations about possible associations between disease and one or more hypothesized risk factors. Determine etiology of disease.	Retrospective - subjects already have disease or condition and are compared with representative group of disease-free persons -controls from the same population.	Useful in studying potential etiologies of rare diseases or diseases with long lag periods between exposure and outcome; Cost and when ethical reasons do not allow RCT.	Looks back – recall bias and incomplete sources for info; ID of comparison group & case selection. Difficult to establish causation.	Recall Bias A statistical relationship between two conditions does not mean that one actually caused the other.
Case Report (single case) or **Case Series** (several similar cases)	Documentation of unique or unusual condition with clinical characteristics.	Present as complete a picture of clinical data, potential exposures or causal factors. Detailed to permit recognition of similar cases by others.	Useful in forming hypotheses and describing clinical experiences; clues for further research; easy and inexpensive.	No statistical validity. Bias in selection of patients; lacks control so not able to generalize.	Patient selection bias; No research design

Table 4-2 Qualitative Research Paradigms

Criteria → / Paradigms (Research Strategy)	Research questions guide (but do not restrict) the inquiry	Methods of data gathering & analysis consistent with philosophical and epistemological traditions from which they are derived and are compatible with the type of question being asked	Methods of data gathering and analysis are rigorously & appropriately applied. Describes: How participants selected. Methods used to generate data. Comprehensiveness of data collection. Procedures for analyzing data	Thoughtful and ethical plan for entering the field of study, establishing and maintaining relationship and exiting the field is illustrated	Conclusions are based upon research results. Data analysis is systematic and meaningful.
Phenomenology Describes lived experiences of individuals as interpreted by the researcher. (Philosophy)	What is the meaning of the phenomenon? What is it like to have a certain experience? Can be related to emotions, relationships, part of an organization or group.	In-depth interviews, written anecdotes, philosophy, poetry or art. Experience provided direction of the study.	Presented examples of research questions.	Identified people, the use of art, poetry, etc.	Reflective description of the experience: "What it felt like to…" Researcher's bias and influence of their own point of view is stated and discussed within the context of the study
Ethnography Used to study people of other cultures. (Cultural anthropology)	What is the nature of this phenomenon? What is the culture of a group of people? Culture may be an ethnic group, organization, program, group of people with common social or health problems.	Participant observation, unstructured interviews, documents, photographs. Researcher learns from participants the meanings they attach to activities, events, behaviors, knowledge, rituals and lifestyle.		Participants and observers of participants	Description of day-to-day events Researcher's bias and influence of their own point of view is stated and discussed within the context of the study
Grounded Theory Discovers basic patterns in social life to generate theories. Used for conceptualizing. (Sociology)	What are the interactions or processes going on? Does not start with a specific research question. Researcher begins study by looking at underlying social and psychological processes that relate to conditions in a particular setting	Taped interviews, participant observation, focus groups, diaries. Studies interactions as they occur naturally.	Researcher identifies key variable that explains what is occurring and further develops emerging theory. Lit review occurs after researcher identifies emerging theory. Data analysis compares emerging theory with existing research (theories).	Key people who play specific roles	Theory development with respect to social and psychological processes. Theory is developed or reformulated from the existing source. Researcher's bias and influence of their own point of view is stated and discussed within the context of the study.

McMaster; http://www.cche.net/usersguides/qualitative.asp
Mita Giacomini, Deborah J. Cook, for the Evidence Based Medicine Working Group. Based on the Users' Guides to Evidence-based Medicine and reproduced with permission from JAMA. (2000 Jul 26;284(4):478-82) Copyright 2000, American Medical Association

Table 4-3. Characteristics of Quantitative and Qualitative Research Approaches[8,9]

	Quantitative		Qualitative
	Experimental	**Non-experimental**	**Non-Experimental**
Purpose and Study Design	Begins with hypothesis and tests cause and effect; variables are defined and manipulated. Answers questions related to therapy and harm in terms of how many or how much; probability sampling allows generalizing findings, uses a deductive process. Double or Single-blinded RCTs or non-blinded RCTs or Controlled Trials	Observational studies used to systematically describe and interpret conditions/relationships that already exist. Examines the association between a particular exposure & a risk factor; or between a disease & hypothesized risk factors. A treatment or intervention is not given. Cohort, Case Control and Case Series or Report studies	Uses a naturalistic approach to answer questions about the meaning, or attitudes, beliefs or behavior or a group or individual; provides explanation & understanding; uses an inductive process; used to generate hypotheses. Phenomenology, Ethnography, & Grounded Theory
Data Collection	Systematic data collection using pre-defined methods of measurement. Often have blinding of examiners to minimize bias when examining experimental and control groups.	Gathers data without giving a treatment or intervening to control variables; clinical exam, survey or questionnaires. Can be collected once or multiple times over time.	Fieldwork to observe people and record in the natural setting. Data collected via focus groups, observation, unstructured interviews, diaries, written anecdotes, philosophy, poetry or art.
Role of Researcher	Tends to remain separate from the subject matter		Tends to be immersed in the subject matter; personal involvement.
Analysis	Analysis occurs after all data is collected. Involves analysis of numerical data that can be combined and manipulated using statistical methods. Results reported using numerical relations and statistical terms.		Analysis takes place concurrently with data collection, and is ongoing. Involves analysis of thoughts or concepts, pictures or objects and categorized into themes. Reported in narrative terms.

Table 4-4. Primary Research Contributes to a Continuum of Knowledge Development & Validation[3]

WATER FLUORIDATION AND ITS RELATIONSHIP TO MOTTLED ENAMEL & CARIES INCIDENCE[5]

CASE REPORT	In 1901 Dr. Frederick S. McKay noted that many of his patients in Colorado Springs, CO, had permanently stained teeth.
HYPOTHESIS	McKay **hypothesized** that the cause was linked to drinking water. Dr. John Eager, who observed United States-bound Italian emigrants from Naples, Italy, noted that when Naples changed its drinking water source, the incidence of stained teeth among infants greatly diminished. In 1925, Dr. McKay noted children who lived in areas where mottled enamel was prevalent had fewer caries.
CLINICAL OBSERVATION	McKay advocated for testing water supplies in communities where mottled enamel disfigured the teeth of children.
EXPERIMENTAL ANIMAL STUDIES	By quantifying fluoride levels in drinking water, 1 ppm was identified as a safe level that did not cause mottling or have toxic effects.
COHORT STUDY	Dr. H. Trendley Dean of the US Public Health Service examined the relationship between fluoride in water supplies and mottled enamel. Dean focused on the link between mottled enamel and the incidence of dental caries and began investigating the effectiveness and safety of fluoridated water. Surveys of school children revealed that those in communities with fluoride had fewer caries than children living in communities with little fluoride in the water.
PROSPECTIVE COMMUNITY-BASED CONTROLLED CLINICAL TRIAL	In 1945, the Grand Rapids fluoridation project began, which confirmed that 1 ppm fluoride significantly lowered the incidence of dental caries without causing mottled enamel or other side effects.

RESEARCH REALITY
(value of a case report)

A case report of clinical observations, one of the lowest levels of evidence, led to the development of hypotheses that were tested and validated through more rigorously designed scientific studies and appropriately designed controlled clinical trials.

THE CONTINUUM OF KNOWLEDGE

The body of evidence evolves over time as more research is conducted. The challenge in using EBDM arises when there is only one research study available on a particular topic. Although the highest level of evidence should be used to support clinical decision making, it also is important to recognize that there may not be a RCT to help answer the question. Lower levels of "evidence" may be useful in contributing to the body of knowledge, as illustrated in Table 4-4, the Continuum of Knowledge Development regarding water fluoridation.

CONCLUSION

As EBDM becomes standard practice, professionals must become good consumers of the scientific literature. To do so requires understanding the different types of research designs used to answer specific questions, and which designs provide the higher levels of evidence. This allows clinicians to better judge the validity of reported findings and to decide if they are relevant to caring for their patient.

Chapter 4 Assignments - Understanding Levels of Evidence: Primary Research Designs

1. **Review the Guide to Research Methods, The Evidence Pyramid** –
    Graphically displays relationship of Research Study Designs and Levels of Evidence.
    Access via https://library.downstate.edu/EBM2/2100.htm

    Review and learn the different research designs and how they relate to Levels of
    Evidence. Focus on the overall learning objectives for this course, which are to:
    *   Explain the research design for each level of evidence: RCT, Cohort Study, Case
        Control Study, Case Reports/Series, Systematic Reviews and Meta-Analyses
    *   Identify the characteristics of each research design, e.g., prospective,
        retrospective, experimental, observational

2. **Watch the NBC News story on Dental X-rays and Meningiomas**
    www.nbcnews.com/video/dental-x-rays-may-raise-risk-of-brain-tumor-44453955975

3. **Complete Exercise 1 on Study Design Characteristics**

4. **Answer the following Critical Thinking Questions:**
    a. Explain the difference between experimental and non-experimental research.
    b. Discuss how qualitative research can complement quantitative findings.
    c. Describe how each research study design contributes to a continuum of
        knowledge and varying levels of evidence.
    d. Identify how bias can influence the results of a study.

5. **Answer the following Self-Reflection Questions:**
    a. What was the one most useful thing you learned in this chapter?
    b. List 2 ways you think you have developed or grown as a result of this chapter?
    c. What problems did you encounter in this chapter, and what if anything, still
        needs further clarification?
    d. What assignment of this chapter was most helpful in learning research design
        and understanding their relationship to levels of evidence?

Exercise 1 - Study Design Characteristics

Identify whether the described study design is quantitative, qualitative, experimental, non-experimental, prospective or retrospective. Please check all that apply.

1. Cohort Study

Check all that apply:

☐ Quantitative   ☐ Experimental   ☐ Prospective

☐ Qualitative   ☐ Non-experimental   ☐ Retrospective

2. Randomized Controlled Trial

Check all that apply:

☐ Quantitative   ☐ Experimental   ☐ Prospective

☐ Qualitative   ☐ Non-experimental   ☐ Retrospective

3. Case Control Study

Check all that apply:

☐ Quantitative   ☐ Experimental   ☐ Prospective

☐ Qualitative   ☐ Non-experimental   ☐ Retrospective

4. Ethnography

Check all that apply:

☐ Quantitative   ☐ Experimental   ☐ Prospective

☐ Qualitative   ☐ Non-experimental   ☐ Retrospective

5. Controlled Trial

Check all that apply:

☐ Quantitative   ☐ Experimental   ☐ Prospective

☐ Qualitative   ☐ Non-experimental   ☐ Retrospective

References

1.   Manolio T. Design and Conduct of Observational Studies and Clinical Trials. In: Gallin J, editor. Principles and Practice of Clinical Research. Academic Press, Elsevier, 2002:187-206.

2.   Claus Eb, Calvocoressi L, Bondy ML, Schildkraut JM, Wiemels JL, Wrensch M. Dental x-rays and risk of meningioma. Cancer, 2012 Sep 15;118(18):4530-7.

3.   National Institute of Dental and Craniofacial Research National Institutes of Health. The story of fluoridation. Accessed 1-27-19.
     https://www.nidcr.nih.gov/health-info/fluoride/the-story-of-fluoridation

4.   Davis J, Chesney P, Wand P. Toxic shock syndrome: Epidemiologic features, recurrence, risk factors, and prevention. N Engl J Med, 1980;303:1429.

5.   Centers for Disease Control. Pneumocystis pneumonia - Los Angeles. MMWR 1981; 30:250.

6.   Giacomini M, Cook DJ. Qualitative Research, Chapter 13.5, In User's Guide to the Medical Literature, 3rd Ed. JAMA evidence Copyright 2015, American Medical Association. Accessed 1-27-19.
     http://jamaevidence.mhmedical.com/content.aspx?bookid=847&sectionid=69031484

7.   Horowitz AM, Canto MT, Child WL. Maryland adults' perspectives on oral cancer prevention and early detection. JADA 2002;133:1061.

8.   Giacomini M, Cook D. User's Guides to the Medical Literature: XXIII. Qualitative Research in Health Care A. Are the Results of the Study Valid? JAMA, 2000;284(3):357-362.

9.   Giacomini M, Cook D. User's Guides to the Medical Literature: XXIII. Qualitative Research in Health Care B. What Are the Results and How Do They Help Me Care for My Patients? JAMA, 2000; 284(4):478-482.

CHAPTER

5

UNDERSTANDING LEVELS OF EVIDENCE:
SECONDARY RESEARCH DESIGN

SECONDARY RESEARCH

Content Outline:
Systematic Reviews & Meta-Analysis
Translating Research into Practice
  • Systems-Clinical Decision Support
  • Guidelines
  • Synopses-Critical Summaries/CATS
Evidence Information Sources
Type of Question & Study Design
Conclusion
Assignments
References

Learning Objectives:
Upon completion of this chapter readers will be able to
1. Explain the difference between primary and secondary research
2. Identify distinguishing characteristics of different sources of secondary research
3. Understand the relationship of secondary research to their corresponding levels of evidence
4. Discuss the hierarchy of evidence information sources
5. Identify types of studies most appropriate to type of question asked

Suggested Assignments:
E1: Study Design Identification
E2: PICO Question & Type of Study
Critical Thinking Questions
Self-Reflection Questions

As evidence-based practice has expanded, so have the resources that provide pre-appraised evidence and critical summaries of that evidence. This chapter reviews secondary sources of evidence and their translation for use in clinical practice. A second hierarchy consisting of levels of evidence information sources is introduced along with corresponding websites that can be explored.

DDS/DMD CODA STANDARDS
EDUCATIONAL ENVIRONMENT, Scientific Discovery and the Integration of Knowledge: the capacity to think scientifically and to apply the scientific method is critical if students are to analyze and solve oral health problems, understand research, and practice evidence-based dentistry.
Critical Thinking, 2-10 Graduates must be competent in the use of critical thinking and problem-solving, including their use in the comprehensive care of patients, scientific inquiry and *research methodology.*
Clinical Sciences, 2-22 Graduates must be competent to access, critically appraise, apply, and communicate scientific and lay literature as it relates to providing evidence-based patient care. Intent: The education program should introduce students to the basic principles of clinical and translational research, including how such research is conducted, evaluated, applied, and explained to patients.

DH CODA STANDARDS
Critical Thinking, 2-22: Graduates must be competent in the evaluation of current scientific literature.

SYNOPSES OF SYSTEMATIC REVIEWS AND INDIVIDUAL STUDIES Critical Summaries

Ideally, practitioners want to be able to quickly access new research that is valid, easy to read, and has been objectively pre-appraised. Over the last decade, how research is presented has evolved to include a very useful form of evidence for practitioners.   A Synopsis or critically appraised summary of secondary (or primary) research is 1-2 pages. It includes a summary of the systematic review (or original individual study) and an expert commentary. The commentary typically includes three components: 1. A critique of the strength and weakness of the methodology of MA/SR (or individual study); 2. A critique of the evidence; and, 3. The practical application of the research to practice along with any concerns or precautions

These critical summaries are useful when nothing exists at the CDSS or Guideline level.[2] Many evidence-based resources have been and are continuing to be developed by evidence-based groups for clinicians in order to facilitate the integration of evidence into their clinical decision-making. This synopsis allows the reader to decide in a few minutes if the evidence is relevant and applicable.

A critically appraised topic (CAT) is a concise one page summary of the best available evidence, created to answer a specific clinical question. A CAT looks like a mini version of a systematic review and usually contains: (Sackett reference)
* a clearly stated clinical/PICO question
* a specific, reproducible search strategy
* a brief description of included articles
* an evidence table of the limitations of included studies
* implications for practice and
* a reference list

EVIDENCE INFORMATION SOURCES

Evidence Information Sources, outlined in the previous section and illustrated in Figure 5-1, are not accessible from a single source or database. It is necessary to know where these sources are located in order to use them in practice. Knowing where to find the **CDSS**, **Guidelines** and **Synopses** are important so that relevant evidence is efficiently accessed from a search. Some of the sites that are highlighted contain multiple tiers of evidence sources. A listing of some pre-appraised evidence resources can be found in Table 5-1.

FINDING COMPUTERIZED DECISION SUPPORT SYSTEMS
External searching of drug databases using individual specific information can assist in identifying and preventing potential harmful situations. Two drug database examples are Lexi-Comp (lexi.com), and Natural Standard (naturalstandard.com) for herbal supplements and complimentary medicine. Although not electronically based, the ADA's Center for EBD provides chair-side support tools related to practice guidelines in several areas of prevention and including non-surgical periodontal treatment. **(ebd.ada.org/en/evidence/guidelines)**

CRITICAL SUMMARY COMMENTARY:

Typically includes three components:

1. A critique of the strength and weakness of the methodology of MA/SR (or individual study)

2. A critique of the evidence

3. The practical application of the research to practice along with any concerns or precautions

---

Dental students, at the University of Texas Health Science Center, prepare a critical appraisal on a specific clinical topic for their CAT (Critically Appraised Topics) Library, now available at **cats.uthscsa.edu**.

Table 5-1. Evidence Information Sources

SYSTEMS: Clinical Decision Support Systems: Interactive Drug Databases

Lexi-Comp, Inc. Comprehensive drug database; Interactions	lexi.com
Natural Standard – Integrative Medicine with EB Grading system	naturalstandard.com

GUIDELINES

American Academy of Pediatric Dentistry (AAPD)	aapd.org/policies
American Academy of Periodontology	perio.org/resources-products/clinical-scientific-papers.html
ADA Clinical Recommendations	ebd.ada.org/en/evidence/guidelines
ADHA, Position Papers and Consensus Statements	adha.org/resources
American Heart Association	professional.americanheart.org
Centers for Disease Control and Prevention	cdc.gov/OralHealth/index.html
PubMed (Filter to Practice Guideline)	pubmed.gov
Scottish Intercollegiate Guidelines Network	sign.ac.uk/our-guidelines.html
Canadian Dental Association	cda-adc.ca/en/about/position_statements/
Canadian Dental Hygiene Association	cdha.ca (Profession Tab, Position Papers)

SYNOPSES OF SYSTEMATIC REVIEWS (CRITICAL SUMMARIES)

ADA Center for Evidence-based Dentistry	ebd.ada.org
PubMed (Look for **Comment in** under the abstract)	pubmed.gov
Evidence Based Dentistry Journal	nature.com/ebd
Journal of Evidence-Based Dental Practice	jebdp.com
Trip Database	tripdatabase.com

SYSTEMATIC REVIEWS

ADA Center for Evidence-based Dentistry	ebd.ada.org
Cochrane Database of Systematic Reviews	cochranelibrary.com
PubMed (Filter to Systematic Reviews)	pubmed.gov
Evidence Based Dentistry journal	nature.com/ebd
Journal of Evidence-Based Dental Practice	jebdp.com
Trip Database	tripdatabase.com

SYNOPSES OF INDIVIDUAL STUDIES

PubMed (Look for **Comment in** under the abstract)	pubmed.gov
Evidence Based Dentistry	nature.com/ebd
Journal of Evidence-Based Dental Practice	jebdp.com

ORIGINAL STUDIES

PubMed	pubmed.gov
Journal Publications	access association & publisher websites

FINDING GUIDELINES

Clinical practice guidelines related to dental and dental hygiene practice can be found on the websites of their professional organizations, such as the American Academy of Pediatric Dentistry (AAPD), **aapd.org/policies**, the American Academy of Periodontology (AAP), **perio.org/members/practice-management-resources**, the American Association of Endodontists (AAE), **aae.org/guidelines**, and the American Dental Hygienists' Association (ADHA), **adha.org**.

ADA CENTER FOR EBD – Resources that help dental practitioners integrate clinically relevant scientific evidence at the point of care including quick access to oral health clinical practice guidelines, systematic reviews from PubMed on oral health topics, and critical summaries. **ebd.ada.org/en/evidence/guidelines**

Examples include guidelines on:

Oral Cancer
Sealants
Topical Fluoride
Fluoride Toothpaste for Young Children
Nonsurgical Treatment of Chronic Periodontitis
Non-restorative Treatments for Carious Lesions
Evaluation of potentially malignant disorders in the oral cavity
Prosthetic Joint Premedication
Fluoride Supplements
Non-fluoride Caries Preventive Agents
Reconstituting Infant Formula
Infective Endocarditis

PRACTICE SKILLS:

Can you find a guideline, synopsis or systematic review about the treatment of burning mouth syndrome for your patient Nathan?

Search three different sources of evidence from Table 5-1. for Nathan.

ADA. Center for Evidence–Based Dentistry™

Clinical Practice Guidelines

Clinical practice guidelines are the strongest resources to aid dental professionals in clinical decision making and help incorporate evidence gained through scientific investigation into patient care. Guidelines include recommendation statements intended to optimize patient care that are informed by a systematic review of evidence and an assessment of the benefits and harms of alternative care options.

TRIP DATABASE - (Translating research into practice), indexes content from several other databases and provides access to clinical practice guidelines, systematic reviews and critical summaries, and primary research. The clinical search engine is designed to allow users to quickly and easily find a high-quality research evidence to support their practice. (See Figures 5-4 through 5-6) **tripdatabase.com**

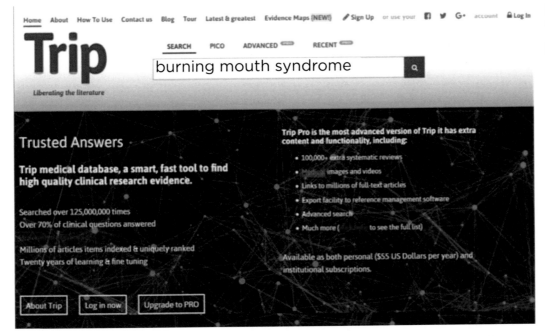

**Figure 5-4.
Trip Database
Homepage**

NHS - An online resource tool kit from the United Kingdom with information for patients and professionals. All health information on the site is evidence-based and peer-reviewed. The Health A-Z section explains more than 800 conditions and treatments in plain language through words, pictures and video. It provides access to clinical practice guidelines and multiple resources. **nhs.uk**

NATIONAL GUIDELINE CLEARINGHOUSE - an initiative of the Agency for Healthcare Research and Quality (AHRQ) that provides health professionals, an accessible mechanism for obtaining objective, detailed information on clinical practice guidelines and to further their dissemination, implementation, and use. **guideline.gov**

FINDING SYNOPSES-CRITICAL SUMMARIES OR CRITICALLY APPRAISED TOPICS (CATS)

There are two evidence-based dentistry journals that provide synopses or critical summaries of both pre-appraised evidence (MAs/SRs) and individual research studies. These EBD journals are Evidence Based Dentistry **nature.com/ebd** and the Journal of Evidence-Based Dental Practice **jebdp.com**. In addition to these two dental journals, many of the general dentistry, dental hygiene, and specialty organization journals are publishing MAs, SRs and critical summaries.

When critically appraised topics, CATs are published in an indexed journal, they can be found through searching PubMed.gov as well.

To begin, type your key words or problem and hit return. Along the left margin you will see color bars that represent the type of study, e.g., secondary evidence, primary research, etc., with the key listed in the right column. To have all secondary evidence listed first, click on All Secondary Evidence. This will reorder the results so that secondary evidence appears first (green color).

Figure 5-5. Trip Database Original Search without Sorting

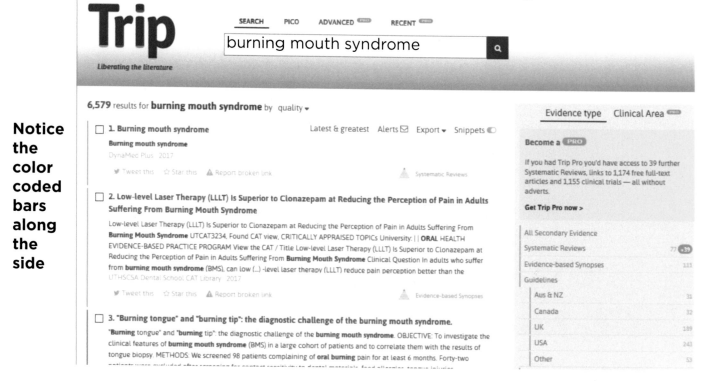

Notice the color coded bars along the side

Figure 5-6. Trip Database Search After Sorting by All Secondary Evidence

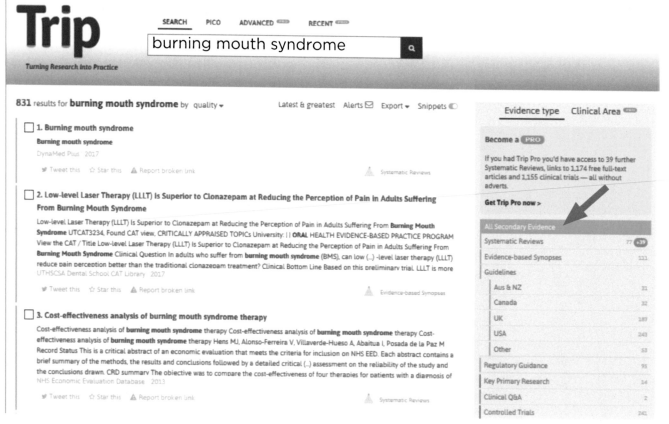

FINDING SYSTEMATIC REVIEWS

THE COCHRANE LIBRARY

The Cochrane Collaboration is an international, independent, non-profit organization comprised of more than 37,000 contributors from more than 130 countries dedicated to producing systematic reviews as a reliable and relevant source of evidence about the effects of health care to support informed decisions across all areas of health care, **cochrane.org**. Rigorous methods and dedication to update their work is has earned the reputation as the international gold standard for high quality trusted information. The Cochrane Oral Health Group is one of 52 groups (**ohg.cochrane.org**). All Cochrane Review groups have an obligation to update the review every two to four years to account for new evidence. The results of their work are housed in the Cochrane Library, **cochranelibrary.com.** (See Figures 5-7 & 8)

Figure 5-7. Cochrane Oral Health Homepage

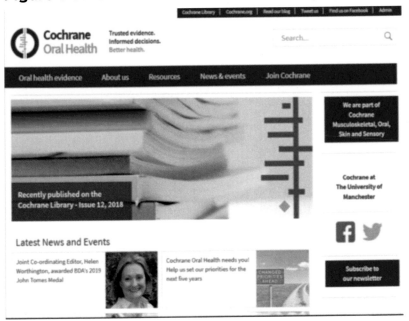

Figure 5-8.
Cochrane Oral Health
Topics

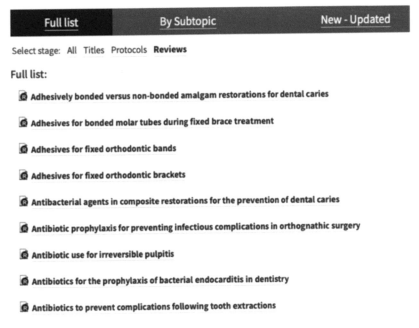

Full list	By Subtopic	New - Updated

Select stage: All Titles Protocols **Reviews**

Full list:

🔹 **Adhesively bonded versus non-bonded amalgam restorations for dental caries**

🔹 **Adhesives for bonded molar tubes during fixed brace treatment**

🔹 **Adhesives for fixed orthodontic bands**

🔹 **Adhesives for fixed orthodontic brackets**

🔹 **Antibacterial agents in composite restorations for the prevention of dental caries**

🔹 **Antibiotic prophylaxis for preventing infectious complications in orthognathic surgery**

🔹 **Antibiotic use for irreversible pulpitis**

🔹 **Antibiotics for the prophylaxis of bacterial endocarditis in dentistry**

🔹 **Antibiotics to prevent complications following tooth extractions**

FINDING SYSTEMATIC REVIEWS

THE COCHRANE LIBRARY

The Cochrane Collaboration is an international, independent, non-profit organization comprised of more than 37,000 contributors from more than 130 countries dedicated to producing systematic reviews as a reliable and relevant source of evidence about the effects of health care to support informed decisions across all areas of health care, **cochrane.org**. Rigorous methods and dedication to update their work is has earned the reputation as the international gold standard for high quality trusted information. The Cochrane Oral Health Group is one of 52 groups (**ohg.cochrane.org**). All Cochrane Review groups have an obligation to update the review every two to four years to account for new evidence. The results of their work are housed in the Cochrane Library, **cochranelibrary.com.**

TYPE OF QUESTION AND STUDY DESIGN

Correctly identifying the type of study most appropriate to answer the clinical/PICO question is an important skill to develop. This guides the clinician to access the appropriate evidence when searching the healthcare literature. For example, identifying the best strategy for managing an endodontic lesion is a treatment question. It is important to know that for a treatment question, MA or SR of RCTs would be the highest level of research on the endodontic treatment being considered. If none if these were available, then the next best evidence would be from a well-conducted individual RCT.

However, when the focus of the question is on the degree to which a test is reliable, such as for detection of oral cancer, then it is a question of diagnosis. In this case the highest level of evidence would be provided by a MA or SR of controlled trials that are studies in which the outcomes of a new diagnostic test are compared with the outcomes of the gold standard test. In this case, the same lesion in the mouth is evaluated using both tests. And again, if a MA or SR were not available, the next highest level would be an individual controlled trial. Table 5-2 illustrates the relationship between the type of question and levels of evidence and study design.

CONCLUSION

Understanding this model and the processing of evidence from primary studies to computerized decision support systems that link an individual patient's characteristics to the most current relevant research about their problem, allows clinicians to become more proficient in finding the highest levels of evidence to answer their clinical questions.

Table 5-2. Type of Question Related to Levels of Evidence and Study Design[6-8]

Type of Question	Type of Study or Methodology of Choice	Question Focus	Why Study?	Example Questions
Therapy/ Prevention	**Systematic Review with Meta-analysis (MA) or Systematic Review without MA (SR) of RCT's** **Single Randomized Controlled Trial** **SR of Cohort Studies**	Study effect of therapy or test on real patients; allows for comparison between intervention and control groups for a particular condition. Largest volume of EB literature.	To select treatments, if any, that do more good than harm (improve function, avoid adverse events) that are worth the effort and cost.	Do sealed permanent first molars need less restorative treatment than unsealed permanent first molars?
Diagnosis	**MA or SR of Controlled Trials** **Single Controlled Trial** (Prospective-compare tests with a reference or "gold" standard test) **Prospective Cohort study**	Measures reliability of a particular diagnostic measure/ test for a disease against the "gold standard" diagnostic measure for the same disease. Sensitivity and specificity of the measures are compared.	To select and interpret diagnostic methods or tests. To determine the degree to which a test is reliable and useful; establish the power of an intervention to differentiate between those with and without a target condition or disease.	How reliable is the _____ saliva test as compared to current caries activity for predicting future caries activity?
Etiology, Causation, Harm	**MA or SR of Cohort Studies** **Single Cohort Study** (Prospective data collection with formal control group) **Case Controlled Study**	Compares a group exposed to a particular agent with an unexposed group. Important for understanding prevention and control of disease.	To identify causes of a disease or condition including iatrogenic forms. To determine relationships between risk factors, potentially harmful agents, and possible causes of a disease or condition.	Does smoking influence vertical alveolar bone loss?
Prognosis	**MA or SR of Inception Cohort Studies** (Follow patients from the onset of a disease or disorder.) **Cohort Study**	Follows progression of a group with particular disease and compares with a group without the disease. Groups must be as similar as possible and must have good follow-up>80% of each group.	To estimate clinical course or progression of a disease or condition over time and anticipate likely complications (and prevent them).	What patient and implant characteristics influence the survival of dental implants?

Chapter 5 Assignments - Understanding Levels of Evidence: Secondary Research Designs

1. Complete the following Exercises – see following pages
- Exercise 1. Study Design Identification
- Exercise 2. Type Of Study & Database Selection Exercise- Identify Research

2. Answer the following Critical Thinking Questions:
a. Explain the difference between primary and secondary research.

b. Discuss how clinical practice guidelines and critical summaries can facilitate the transfer of research to clinical practice.

c. Discuss why it is important to look at different databases when conducting a search.

3. Answer the following Self-Reflection Questions:
a. What was the one most useful thing you learned in this chapter?

b. List 2 ways you think you have developed or grown as a result of this chapter?

c. What problems did you encounter in this chapter, and what if anything, still needs further clarification?

d. What assignment of this chapter was most helpful in learning research design and understanding their relationship to levels of evidence?

e. Describe your experience exploring the evidende information sources.

Exercise 1 - Study Design Identification

Identify the study design described

1. **Randomly assigned subjects, randomly assigned treatments, experimental and control groups**

   ☐_____Meta-Analysis   ☐_____Systematic Review (SR)   ☐_____Randomized Controlled Trial

   ☐_____Clinical Trial   ☐_____Practice Guideline   ☐_____Critical Summary of SR

   ☐_____Cohort Study   ☐_____Case Control Study   ☐_____Case Series or Case Report

   ☐_____Review   ☐_____Critical Summary of an Individual Study

2. **Analysis of pooled data from a compilation of individual studies**

   ☐_____Meta-Analysis   ☐_____Systematic Review (SR)   ☐_____Randomized Controlled Trial

   ☐_____Clinical Trial   ☐_____Practice Guideline   ☐_____Critical Summary of SR

   ☐_____Cohort Study   ☐_____Case Control Study   ☐_____Case Series or Case Report

   ☐_____Review   ☐_____Critical Summary of an Individual Study

3. **A retrospective study that observes possible associations between a disease and one or more hypothesized risk factors**

   ☐_____Meta-Analysis   ☐_____Systematic Review (SR)   ☐_____Randomized Controlled Trial

   ☐_____Clinical Trial   ☐_____Practice Guideline   ☐_____Critical Summary of SR

   ☐_____Cohort Study   ☐_____Case Control Study   ☐_____Case Series or Case Report

   ☐_____Review   ☐_____Critical Summary of an Individual Study

4. **Observes associations between risk factors and the development of a disease**

   ☐_____Meta-Analysis   ☐_____Systematic Review (SR)   ☐_____Randomized Controlled Trial

   ☐_____Clinical Trial   ☐_____Practice Guideline   ☐_____Critical Summary of SR

   ☐_____Cohort Study   ☐_____Case Control Study   ☐_____Case Series or Case Report

   ☐_____Review   ☐_____Critical Summary of an Individual Study

5. **Reports the treatment of a single patient or several patients with the same condition**

   ☐_____Meta-Analysis   ☐_____Systematic Review (SR)   ☐_____Randomized Controlled Trial

   ☐_____Clinical Trial   ☐_____Practice Guideline   ☐_____Critical Summary of SR

   ☐_____Cohort Study   ☐_____Case Control Study   ☐_____Case Series or Case Report

   ☐_____Review   ☐_____Critical Summary of an Individual Study

6. **Synthesis of findings from individual studies on the same topic**

   ☐_____Meta-Analysis   ☐_____Systematic Review (SR)   ☐_____Randomized Controlled Trial

   ☐_____Clinical Trial   ☐_____Practice Guideline   ☐_____Critical Summary of SR

   ☐_____Cohort Study   ☐_____Case Control Study   ☐_____Case Series or Case Report

   ☐_____Review   ☐_____Critical Summary of an Individual Study

7. **Systematically developed statements about appropriate health care for specific clinical circumstances**

   ☐_____Meta-Analysis   ☐_____Systematic Review (SR)   ☐_____Randomized Controlled Trial

   ☐_____Clinical Trial   ☐_____Practice Guideline   ☐_____Critical Summary of SR

   ☐_____Cohort Study   ☐_____Case Control Study   ☐_____Case Series or Case Report

   ☐_____Review   ☐_____Critical Summary of an Individual Study

Exercise 2 - Type of Question & Type of Studies

Research Designs and Sources of Evidence

1. Case Control Study
2. Case Report
3. Cohort Study
4. Controlled Trial

5. Critical Summary of MA or SR
6. Critical Summary of RCT
7. Inception Cohort Study
8. Meta-Analysis (MA)

9. Randomized Controlled Trial
10. Practice Guideline
11. Systematic Review (SR)

Review the following PICO questions and identify the Type of Question being asked and determine from the above list the appropriate Primary Research Design and the first three Secondary Sources of Evidence in order from highest (#1) to lowest (#3) level of evidence. Write the number (1-11) of the research design/source of evidence in the spaces provided.

1. For adult patients with recurrent aphthous ulcers (cold sores), will a daily zinc supplement compared to a 0.12% chlorhexidine daily rinse more effectively reduce the frequency of outbursts?

    Type of Question: ☐ Therapy/ Prevention ☐ Diagnosis ☐ Etiology, Causation, Harm ☐ Prognosis

    Primary Research Design: _____ (write the number of the research design from list)

    Secondary Source: (Highest) 1._____   2._____   3._____ (Lowest)

2. For adults with dental implants, will diabetes significantly decrease the longevity of the implants?

    Type of Question: ☐ Therapy/ Prevention ☐ Diagnosis ☐ Etiology, Causation, Harm ☐ Prognosis

    Primary Research Design: _____ (write the number of the research design from list)

    Secondary Source: (Highest) 1._____   2._____   3._____ (Lowest)

3. For a patient with a prosthetic joint placed 3 months ago, should prophylactic antibiotic coverage be prescribed prior to undergoing dental procedures to prevent infection?

    Type of Question: ☐ Therapy/ Prevention ☐ Diagnosis ☐ Etiology, Causation, Harm ☐ Prognosis

    Primary Research Design: _____ (write the number of the research design from list)

    Secondary Source: (Highest) 1._____   2._____   3._____ (Lowest)

4. For a patient with periapical bone lesions, will cone beam computed tomography (CBCT), as compared to traditional intraoral radiographs, be more accurate in assessing apical bone destruction?

    Type of Question: ☐ Therapy/ Prevention ☐ Diagnosis ☐ Etiology, Causation, Harm ☐ Prognosis

    Primary Research Design: _____ (write the number of the research design from list)

    Secondary Source: (Highest) 1._____   2._____   3._____ (Lowest)

References

1. Mulrow C. Rationale for systematic reviews. BMJ 1994;309(6954):597-599.

2. DiCenso A, Bayley L, Haynes RB. Accessing preappraised evidence: fine-tuning the 5S model into a 6S Model, editorial. ACP Journal Club, 15 September 2009, 151(3):JC3-2 – JC3-3.

3. Oshreroff JA, Teich JM, Middleton BF, Steen EB, Wright A, Detmer DE. A Roadmap for National Action on Clinical Decision Support, June13, 2006. Accessed 01-27-19.
    Available at: https://www.amia.org/sites/default/files/files_2/A-Roadmap-for-National-Action-on-Clinical-Decision-Support-June132006.pdf

4. Montini T, Schenkel AB, Shelley DR. Feasibility of a computerized clinical decision support system for treating tobacco use in dental clinics. J Dent Educ, 2013 Apr:77(4):458-62.

5. Committee on Quality of Health Care in America, IOM. Crossing the Quality Chasm: A New Health System for the 21st Century. Washington DC: The National Academy of Sciences, 2000.

6. OCEBM Levels of Evidence Working Group. The Oxford 2011 Levels of Evidence. Oxford Centre for Evidence-Based Medicine. Accessed 01-27-19.
    Available at: http://www.cebm.net/index.aspx?o=5653

7. Guyatt G, Rennie D, Meade MO, Cook DJ. Users' Guide to Medical Literature: A Manual for Evidence-Based Clinical Practice, 2nd Edition, JAMA, Chicago: McGraw Hill, 2008.

8. Haynes R, Wilczynski N, McGibbon A, Walker C, Sinclair J. Developing optimal search strategies for detecting clinically sound studies in MEDLINE. J Am Med Inform Assoc, 1994;1(6):447-458.

NOTES

CHAPTER

6

FINDING EVIDENCE: KNOWING HOW TO LOOK

Skill 2. ACCESS:
Conducting a computerized search with maximum efficency for finding the best external evidence with which to answer the question

Content Outline:
Searching Methods
PubMed Key Features
  • MeSH terms
  • Boolean Operators
  • Filters: Inclusion & Exclusion Criteria
  • Clinical Queries
  • Printing the Search Strategy
Conclusion
Assignments
References

Learning Objectives:
Upon completion of this chapter, readers will be able to

1. Explain types of research found using PubMed
2. Discuss key searching components of PubMed
3. Identify MeSH terms for a PICO question
4. Compare Advanced and Clinical Queries search
5. Efficiently use PubMed to find evidence to answer a PICO question

Suggested Assignments:
Dentalcare.com searching course
PubMed Tutorials
Search using Nathan Case
Critical Thinking Questions
Self-Reflection Questions

The purpose of this chapter is to discuss online scientific databases and demonstrate an efficient computerized search. This step in the evidence-based process facilitates developing a conscious, strategic search of the existing body of evidence in order to ensure the best, most relevant research is found. The oral health care provider has an ethical, legal and professional responsibility to make certain the best information is found to advise or treat a patient. As one of the largest scientific databases, PubMed has been selected to demonstrate searching. Also, it provides free access to abstracts and some full-text articles.

Two assignments that are helpful to complete prior to or in conjunction with this chapter are:

Strategies for Searching the Literature Using PubMed at dentalcare.com

PubMed Tutorials at learn.nlm.nih.gov/documentation/training-packets/T0042010P/

DDS/DMD CODA STANDARDS
EDUCATIONAL ENVIRONMENT, Critical Thinking: The components of critical thinking are: the application of logic and accepted intellectual standards to reasoning; the ability to access and evaluate evidence... and develop students who are able to gather and assess relevant information...
Clinical Sciences, 2-22 Graduates must be competent to access, critically appraise, apply and communicate scientific and lay literature as it relates to providing evidence-based patient care.

DH CODA STANDARDS
Critical Thinking, 2-23: Graduates must be competent in problem solving strategies related to comprehensive patient care and management of patients.

SEARCHING METHODS

Once a good clinical question has been formulated using the PICO process, the second step in using EBDM is to conduct a computerized search to find the best external evidence for answering the question. This type of search requires a shift in thinking. Often, especially now with fast web-based search engines and smartphones with "intelligence assistants," health professionals look for "something" on a topic, a quick answer, or for "everything." Finding relevant evidence requires conducting a focused search of peer-reviewed professional literature based on the appropriate research methodology. This forces the clinician to know where to look and how to look for primary and secondary research.

Knowing how to find the research is important so that key articles and evidence are accessed efficiently from each search. This chapter compliments the online course, "Searching the Literature Using PubMed" on Dentalcare.com. PubMed is selected because it provides free access to MEDLINE, the largest scientific database, and many of the other databases draw their information from PubMed or refer back to PubMed.

PubMed KEY FEATURES

Searching for evidence requires new information retrieval skills in order to take full advantage of the capabilities that PubMed and other databases provide. Understanding how these are structured, their language and searching rules increases your abilities and success in finding relevant evidence. As with learning any new skills, efficiently searching for valid evidence using online databases can be frustrating. However, with a little time and practice they can be mastered so that the best evidence can be accessed with maximum efficiency. PubMed is accessed online at **pubmed.gov**. Three imporant resources accessed here are the PubMed tutorials, Clinical Queries and the MeSH database (Figure 6-1).

MeSH MEDICAL SUBJECT HEADINGS (MeSH˚)

The National Library of Medicine uses a special vocabulary of biomedical terms to index primary and secondary research using **Medical Subject Headings (MeSH)**. This allows articles to be searchable according to these specifically defined terms.

The MeSH Database can be accessed from the homepage (Figure 6-1) or at ncbi.nlm.nih.gov/mesh. The database allows users to enter a text word or phrase to display how MEDLINE defines the term, the date it was introduced and any other terms it was indexed as previously. This database has an auto complete feature that offers possible MeSH terms based on what is typed. Typing a term shows a drop down menu with the ability to choose from a list of terms that may be applicable to the search. It also displays how Medline searches for that term by illustrating how it is indexed hierarchically by category (in a MeSH tree) with more specific terms arranged beneath broader terms[1] (Figure 6-2). This is helpful to know when search results are too small because

Figure 6-1 PubMed Homepage

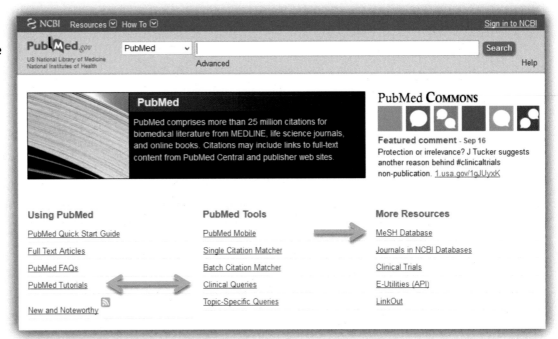

Figure 6-2 Burning Mouth Syndrome MeSH Term, Subheadings, Previous Indexing and Tree

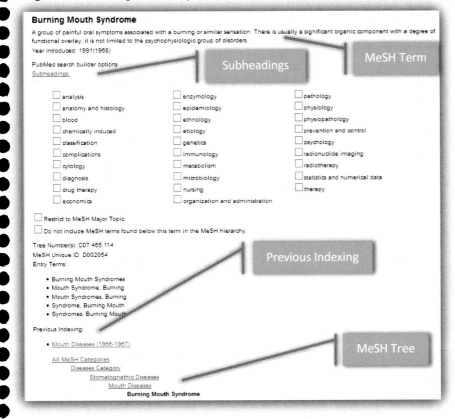

Publication Types, MeSH Terms, Substances

Publication Types
Comparative Study
Research Support, Non-U.S. Gov't

MeSH Terms
Anxiety/complications
Anxiety/drug therapy
Burning Mouth Syndrome/drug therapy*
Burning Mouth Syndrome/etiology
Chi-Square Distribution
Clonazepam/therapeutic use*
Depression/complications
Depression/drug therapy
Diazepam/therapeutic use*
Female
GABA Modulators/therapeutic use*
Humans
Male
Personality Inventory
Questionnaires
Retrospective Studies
Statistics, Nonparametric

Substances
GABA Modulators
Clonazepam
Diazepam

Figure 6-3 MeSH Terms with the Abstract using Drop Down Menu

RESULTS: A total of 71.4 per cent of patients treated with clonazepam had partial or complete resolution of their oral symptoms, while 55.1 per cent of patients treated with diazepam had improvement of their oral symptoms. There was no correlation between underlying anxiety or depression and efficacy of benzodiazepine medication.

CONCLUSIONS: A greater percentage of patients taking clonazepam reported either partial or complete relief of symptoms compared to diazepam. However, the differences were not statistically significant. There was no correlation found between underlying psychopathology and treatment success with benzodiazepines.

PMID: 20415927 [PubMed - indexed for MEDLINE]

Publication Types, MeSH Terms, Substances

using the broader term can help increase the search results. MeSH terms also can be found below each abstract, in the drop down menu Publication Types, MeSH Terms, Substances (Figure 6-3). This can be extremely helpful when relevant research is limited because it tells the searcher how the citation is indexed which can provide additional keywords. These terms can be added to a search to find similar studies and additional evidence.[7]

BOOLEAN OPERATORS

Boolean operators are words used to associate terms. They limit results of a search by allowing the combination of search terms or concepts. PubMed processes Boolean operators from left-to-right. The order of processing can change by nesting an individual concept in parentheses. The terms inside the parentheses will be processed as a unit and then incorporated into the overall strategy. This is similar to nesting numbers in a math problem: (3X2) + (7X4) vs. (3 X 2 + 7 X 4).

The three Boolean operators are AND, OR and NOT, and must be capitalized when using them on PubMed.[2] An example of a search using nesting is:

(Tooth Bleaching NOT Toothpaste) OR (Whitening Strips AND carbamide peroxide) .

Figure 6-4
Boolean Operator **AND**

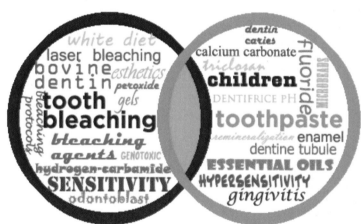

The **AND** operator is used to retrieve results that contain **all** of the search terms in a citation. **AND combines only sets that contain BOTH terms.** The default operator used in PubMed is AND. If you do not include Boolean operators in your search, PubMed will automatically use AND between terms.[2] PubMed looks for keywords in the title, abstract, journal, author, editor or text words.

A search for "Toothpaste AND Tooth Bleaching" will retrieve only citations that reference both toothpaste and tooth bleaching (Figure 6-4).

The **OR** operator **combines citations that have at least one of the terms.** The OR operator is typically used to combine search terms that are related or to broaden a search. This boolean operator typically retrieves more citations because it includes all the results that have the search terms together. (Figure 6-5). An example search is Toothpaste OR Tooth Bleaching.

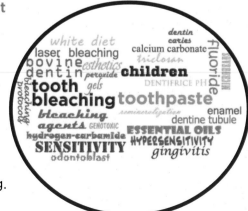

Figure 6-5
Boolean Operator **OR**

The **NOT** operator **excludes the retrieval of terms from search results** (Figure 6-6). However, beware - using the NOT Boolean operator in the search strategy may eliminate relevant citations that contain relevant information.[9] For example, a search for "Tooth Bleaching NOT Toothpaste" excludes results about toothpaste, therefore focusing the results on only Tooth Bleaching that isn't delivered through a toothpaste. So, a relevant study that compared the effectiveness of teeth whitening using whitening strips, whitening gel, and whitening toothpaste would be excluded even though it may answer your question because toothpaste was one of the variables.

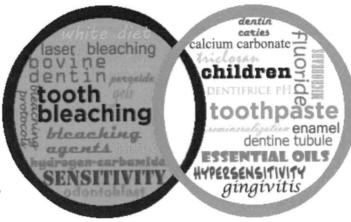

Figure 6-6
Boolean Operator **NOT**

FILTERS (INCLUSION AND EXCLUSION CRITERIA)

The Filters feature allows the user to limit the results of a search to specific fields. The filters can be customized to include criteria not listed in the default table by clicking on Customize. The Article Type filter allows a search to be limited to research methodology, such as Systematic Review, Meta-Analysis, Practice Guideline or Randomized Control Trial. This filter is key to conducting an efficient search and specifically for retrieving the higher levels of evidence. Additional filters include Text Availability, Ages, Language and Journal Categories. The filter choices are conveniently located on the left side bar of the PubMed search screen. To apply a filter to your search, simply click on the desired filter. Once selected these filters remain active for future searches. The selected filters appear above the search results. The most used filters display by default. To show additional filters, click on the link at the bottom of the sidebar to add more options.

Selecting multiple filters from one category will automatically add each selection with the Boolean operator "OR," expanding the search results. For example, using the Article Types filter and selecting Systematic Review, Meta-Analysis, and Practice Guideline will produce results that include all of those methodologies together. Keep in mind that only filters which are valid for your search results will appear. For example, if no Practice Guidelines are in your results, the filter for Practice Guidelines will not appear.[3]

Filters allow the user to limit search results based on inclusion or exclusion criteria. This is important when the PICO question addresses an explicit population such as infant children with baby bottle tooth decay, or teenagers with juvenile diabetes. To find research relevant to that population, use the age range filter.

Exclusion criteria also are helpful in filtering for relevant citations. As explained in the Boolean Operators section, NOT can be used to exclude irrelevant terms. Exclusion criteria are important when search results are large because it helps to reduce results to a manageable size and increase the relevancy of the citations.

CLINICAL QUERIES

A valuable tool for conducting an efficient evidence-based search is the Clinical Queries feature, accessible from the homepage. It supports evidence-based searching by using a specialized algorithm to retrieve the highest levels of evidence on questions of therapy, diagnosis, etiology, prognosis or clinical prediction guides. (Figure 6-7)

Figure 6-7 PubMed Clinical Queries

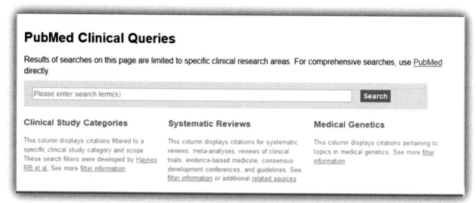

This feature provides a quick check of the literature based on the Type of Question by using specialized, automated filters to retrieve the highest levels of evidence. It allows for fast results on a topic. Clinical Queries has a Systematic Review search, which displays citations for secondary research including systematic reviews, meta-analyses, reviews of clinical trials, evidence-based medicine, consensus development conferences, and guidelines. Searching under the Clinical Study Categories retrieves the highest levels of primary research.

Figure 6-8 Advanced
Search History/Strategy

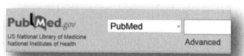

REPRODUCIBLE SEARCH STRATEGY

The advanced search builder in PubMed makes it easy to see the search strategy. The YouTube Tutorial on this page is very helpful in explaining how to use this tool in a search. Clicking on the **Advanced** link under the search bar displays the search strategy (Figure 6-8). This is available to download as an excel spreadsheet or print from the browser.

Save selected abstracts to a file, clipboard or email. **<u>Send to:</u>** displays a pull down menu that allows the user to fill out the form for the appropriate selection. It provides options for the format of the content, whether or not to include MeSH and other data and how many citations to send. Additional comments can be included in an email as well from this pull down menu.

CONCLUSION

Learning the skill to quickly access relevant research studies to answer a specific question takes time and patience. Proficiency comes through practice and experience. The Translating Evidence Into Practice Tool (Table 6-2) provides a framework for conducting a PubMed search.

Table 6-2. Translating Evidence into Practice Tool

Name _____   Topic <u>Burning Mouth Syndrome</u>

1. **Type of study (Article Type) to include in the search:**

   Check all that apply, then number from highest (#1) to lowest level of evidence:

✓__3__Meta-Analysis	✓__4__Systematic Review (SR)	✓__5__Randomized Controlled Trial
☐_____Clinical Trial	✓__1__Practice Guideline	✓__2__Critical Summary of SR
☐_____Cohort Study	☐_____Case Control Study	☐_____Case Series or Case Report
☐_____Review	☐_____Critical Summary of an Individual Study	

2. **List main topics and alternate terms from your PICO question**
   Circle MeSH terms.

Burning mouth syndrome	Elavil®
Tricyclic antidepressants	Amitriptyline
Antidepressive agents	Klonopin®
Benzodiazepines	Chlordiazepoxide
Clonazepam	Librium®

3. **List inclusion criteria-age, language, publication date**

   Human

   English

   List irrelevant terms to exclude

4. **Check the databases to search for evidence**

✓ PubMed/Medline	✓ TRIP Database
✓ National Guideline Clearinghouse	☐ ADHA, Position Papers & Consensus Statements
✓ Cochrane Library	☐ Scottish Intercollegiate Guidelines Network
✓ ADA CEBD	☐ Other:_____

Chapter 6 Assignments - Finding Evidence

1.   Complete the tutorial: **Searching the Literature Using PubMed** accessed at dentalcare.com Focus on the overall learning objectives for this course.

Follow the general Instructions in Chapter 2 (pg 15) **OR** use an Assignment Number provided by the Instructor to access the online course with the following instructions:

1. Go to: http://www.dentalcare.com
2. Register if you already have not done so. You must be registered to take the Quiz at the end of the course and receive a Certificate.
3. Under **Professional Education**, click on **Take a Course**.
4. Scroll down the page to where it says **Students Only** and **enter the assignment number** and click **GO**.
5. Once on the course site, click on **TAKE COURSE NOW**
6. There also is the option to Download the course (pdf) to save for future reference/study.
7. **Upon successful completion of the Quiz, you will be emailed a certificate. Save it for verification.**
   (OPTION: Print it out and bring to class or email to instructor.)

2.   View the following short PubMed tutorials to enhance a PubMed search:

MeSH - youtube.com/watch?v=uyF8uQY9wys
Boolean Logic- nlm.nih.gov/bsd/disted/pubmedtutorial/020_350.html
Filters - youtube.com/watch?v=696R9GbOyvA

3. **Complete Exercise 1 on Searching Practice**

4. **Complete Exercise 2 on Searching Practice**

5. **Answer the following Critical Thinking Questions:**
   a. Why are MeSH terms helpful when searching PubMed/Medline?

   b. Describe one new aspect of PubMed learned after completing the this chapter. How will this help you search for answers to questions more effectively?

   c. Compare and contrast an Advanced search with a Clinical Queries search.

6. **Answer the following Self-Reflection Questions:**
   a. Am I able to find MeSH terms effectively??

   b. Am I able to use each feature of PubMed to create an effective search to answer a PICO question?

   c. Am I able to find the highest level of evidence available using Filters?

   d. What problems did I encounter in this chapter?

   e. What still needs further clarification?

Exercise 1 - Searching Practice

PICO QUESTION:

For a patient with burning mouth syndrome, will tricyclic anti-depressants, compared to benzodiazepines, be more effective in relieving the burning sensation on his lips and tongue?

1. Use Table 6-2 Translating Evidence into Practice Tool to practice searching PubMed for answers to the above PICO question.

2. Use each feature of PubMed to:
   - Find the MeSH terms
   - Use boolean operators to combine terms
   - Filter for highest levels of evidence and
   - Print or save the search strategy.

3. Conduct a search for the same PICO question using the Clinical Queries Feature.

4. Search additional databases (listed in #4 of Table 6-2) for evidence to answer the PICO question for Nathan.

   ✓ PubMed/Medline
   ✓ National Guideline Clearinghouse
   ✓ Cochrane Library
   ✓ ADA CEBD

   ✓ TRIP Database
   ☐ ADHA, Position Papers & Consensus Statements
   ☐ Scottish Intercollegiate Guidelines Network
   ☐ Other:_____

Exercise 2 - Searching Practice

Briefly write about a situation, topic, or patient/ problem for which you do not have answers or need more complete information.

1.   Summarize your topic, situation or patient problem:

2.   Define your PICO Components
        (These should be used to help establish your search strategy)
        Problem:_____
        Intervention:_____
        Comparison: _____
        Outcome:_____

3.   Write out your PICO question using the formula.

4.   Identify the Type of question. **Circle one**:

        Therapy/Prevention   Diagnosis   Etiology, Causation, or Harm   Prognosis

5.   Identify 3 key word/search terms to use for your search on this topic:
                a.
                b.
                c.

6.   Use each feature of PubMed to:
        a.   Identify MeSH terms related to your 3 key search terms

        b.   Write out 2 search strategies using the identified key/MeSH terms and how
                you will combine them using Boolean operators to find an answer to your
                PICO Question:

        c.   Conduct a traditional PubMed search and filter for the highest levels of
                evidence

        d.   Conduct the same search using Clinical Queries

        e.   Identify the article that best answers your question you found using PubMed/
                Clinical Queries.

        (Put complete reference: Authors, Name of Article, Journal name, year, pages)

Exercise 2 - Searching Practice (continued)

7.   Do a search using the Tripdatabase.com.

    a.   What term did you type in on the homepage to begin your search?_____

    b.   How many secondary relevant references did you find? _____

    c.   Were they different than what you found using PubMed? If so, identify one that is different and answers your question (Put complete reference: Authors, Name of Article, Journal name, year, pages).

        _____

        _____

8.   Do a search on the ADA's Center for Evidence-Based Dentistry (ebd.ada.org) Click on Evidence to begin to explore if it has a systematic review or practice guideline related to your topic.

    a.   What term did you type in on the homepage to begin your search?_____

    b.   How many secondary relevant references did you find?_____

    c.   Were they different than what you found using PubMed? If so, identify one that is different and answers your question (Put complete reference: Authors, Name of Article, Journal name, year, pages).

        _____

        _____

9.   Search a professional association site related to your topic, e.g., if you're topic deals with gingivitis go to the AAP website, perio.org and look under Publications, Clinical and Scientific Papers OR if your topic deals with children, go to the AAPD website, aapd.org. See Table 5-1 for a listing of different evidence information sources.

    a.   What website did you search? _____

    b.   Where on the website did you find information?_____

    c.   Identify the process and # of steps you went through to find the information:

        1._____

        2._____

        3._____

        4._____

    d.   How many relevant secondary references did you find?

    e.   Were they different than what you found using PubMed? If so, identify one that is different and answers your question (Put complete reference: Authors, Name of Article, Journal name, year, pages).

    ✓ PubMed/Medline   ✓ TRIP Database

    ✓ National Guideline Clearinghouse   ☐ ADHA, Position Papers & Consensus Statements

    ✓ Cochrane Library   ☐ Scottish Intercollegiate Guidelines Network

    ✓ ADA CEBD   ☐ Other:_____

References

1. National Library of Medicine, NCBI. PubMed. National Library of Medicine, NIH, 2001. PubMed MeSH Browser Tutorial https://www.youtube.com/watch?v=uyF8uQY9wys Accessed: 1/27/19

2. National Library of Medicine, NCBI. PubMed. National Library of Medicine, NIH, 2001. PubMed Boolean Logic https://www.nlm.nih.gov/bsd/disted/pubmedtutorial/020_350.html Accessed 01/27/19

3. National Library of Medicine, NCBI. PubMed. National Library of Medicine, NIH, 2001. PubMed Filters Tutorial https://www.youtube.com/watch?v=696R9GbOyvA Accessed 01/27/19

NOTES

NOTES

CHAPTER

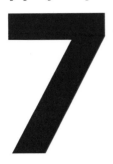

APPRAISING THE SCIENTIFIC LITERATURE

The purpose of this chapter is to discuss critical appraisal criteria and the evaluation tools that simplify the process of determining the credibility and usefulness of the evidence. These tools can be used to assess the methodological quality of a study and assist in making initial judgments. Using these tools will help users determine the validity of the study by examining the strengths and weaknesses of how the study was conducted.

DDS/DMD CODA STANDARDS
EDUCATIONAL ENVIRONMENT, Critical Thinking:
The components of critical thinking are: the application of logic and accepted intellectual standards to reasoning; the ability to access and evaluate evidence...
- Gather and assess relevant information weighing it against extant knowledge and ideas, to interpret information accurately and arrive at well-reasoned conclusions.

Educational Environment, Evidence-based Care: Evidence-based dentistry (EBD) is an approach to oral health care that requires the judicious integration of systematic assessments of clinically relevant scientific evidence.

Clinical Sciences, 2-22 Graduates must be competent to access, critically appraise, apply, and communicate scientific and lay literature as it relates to providing evidence-based patient care.

DH CODA STANDARDS
Critical Thinking, 2-22: Graduates must be competent in the evaluation of current scientific literature.

Critical Thinking, 2-23: Graduates must be competent in problem solving strategies related to comprehensive patient care and management of patients.

KEY QUESTIONS IN APPRAISING THE SCIENTIFIC LITERATURE

PRELIMINARY QUESTIONS

Having an understanding of research design provides the foundation necessary for the critical appraisal process. For many practitioners, the skills for understanding and evaluating research studies are not second nature. In thinking about the methodological quality of an article, some preliminary background questions can be asked to decide what the paper is about.[1]

- First, why was the study conducted and what question was the author addressing? Is there a PICO question or an explicitly stated objective or purpose?
- Next, what type of study was conducted? Is a primary or secondary study described?
- Finally, was the design appropriate to answer the question? For example, if a treatment and placebo are being compared, was an RCT used, or if a new diagnostic instrument is being tested, was a controlled trial conducted? These types of questions will help you get an initial handle on the focus of the study.

Fortunately, evidence-based groups have developed guidelines and tools to assist in critical appraisal of the evidence. These tools consist of a structured series of questions or items that help review the validity of the study. **Validity** is defined by the User's Guides to the Medical Literature as the degree to which a study appropriately answers the question being asked or an instrument measures what it is supposed to measure and performs the functions that it purports to perform.[2]

Reliability refers to the consistency of a set of measurements or a measuring instrument. A test instrument is said to be reliable if it yields consistent results over repeated tests of the same subject under ideal conditions. However, just because a test or instrument is reliable does not mean it is valid.

CRITICAL APPRAISAL QUESTIONS

The Journal of the American Medical Association (JAMA) Series of articles on the Users' Guides to the Medical Literature, prepared by the Evidence-Based Medicine Working Group,[2] serve as the basis for various checklists of critical appraisal questions. One group, the Critical Appraisal Skills Programme (CASP), **casp-uk.net/casp-tools-checklists**, offers online downloadable learning resources including PDF checklists to appraise Systematic Reviews (SRs), Randomized Controlled Trial (RCTs), Cohort studies, Case Control studies, and Diagnostic test studies. The CASP checklists consist of a structured series of YES/Can't Tell/ NO questions that are based on three key questions

1. Are the results of the study valid?
2. What are the results?
3. Will the results help in caring for my patient?

Key questions are important in that they assist practitioners in determining if they can place confidence in the results. For

---

VALIDITY vs. RELIABILITY

Do not confuse validity with reliability.

If an **explorer** is used **to measure pocket depth**, the same results may be obtained over and over and be reliable. Yet, an explorer is not the correct instrument to measure pocket depth so the results are not valid.

When evaluating test instruments, validity is more important than reliability, however to be useful, there must be both reasonable validity and reliability.

example, in reviewing the first question, "<u>Are the Results of the Study Valid?</u>", it's important to know the specific question addressed and if it was reasonable. How patients are recruited, randomly assigned and treated throughout the study indicates if the methods used minimize bias, are reproducible and are appropriate for the question being studied. A subset of more detailed questions exists for each of the three key questions, which further helps determine the validity, results and applicability of the evidence.[2] If answering these questions results in a "No" response, i.e., the study methods are not valid, then there is no point in continuing since the results will not be meaningful. (See Figure 7-1)

Table 7-1 illustrates the three key CASP questions and the related subset of questions for each type of question: Therapy/ Prevention, Diagnosis, Prognosis, and Harm/Etiology/Causation.

APPRAISAL GUIDELINES

In an effort to improve the quality of published research, several international guidelines have been published for the reporting of research studies. These differ from the CASP appraisal tools in that the focus is on what should be included in the publication of the study. They also differ from CASP in that each group has only created a guideline for one specific type of study. For example, the EQUATOR Network publishes the CONSORT statement, (Consolidated Standards of Reporting Trials), which is designed to improve the quality of reporting randomized clinical trials (RCTs), and PRISMA (Preferred Reporting Items for Systematic Reviews and Meta-analyses), guidelines which are designed to improve the reporting of Systematic Reviews (SRs). These guidelines and flow charts help guarantee the integrity of the reported results and also serve as criteria that clinicians can use for evaluating an RCT or SR/MA.

The online version of the CONSORT checklist links to an explanation of each criterion should the user need further information. Unlike CASP forms, which use a YES/Can't Tell/NO format, the CONSORT and PRISMA forms ask the reviewer to list the page number where the information was reported.

The CONSORT statement is available in multiple languages and has been endorsed by over 580 journals, including such prominent medical journals such as The Lancet, Annals of Internal Medicine, the Journal of the American Medical Association and the New England Journal of Medicine (NEJM). Several journals, including the NEJM now request authors to provide a flow diagram in CONSORT format and all of the information required by the CONSORT checklist when reporting on clinical trials. The same requirements are made regarding the reporting of MAs or SRs using the PRISMA flowchart. These requirements assist in standardizing the peer review process and help practitioners understand the experimental process so that they can evaluate the validity of the study and interpret the clinical importance of the overall results.

APPRAISAL or STANDARD FOR REPORTING CHECKLISTS

CASP
Systematic Reviews (SRs), Randomized Controlled Trial (RCTs), Cohort studies, Case Control studies, and Diagnostic test studies.
casp-uk.net/casp-tools-checklists

equator-network.org links to the following checklists

CONSORT
randomized clinical trials (RCTs)

PRISMA
Systematic Reviews and Meta-analyses

STARD
Studies of diagnostic accuracy

STROBE
Observational Studies: Cohort studies, case-control studies, and cross-sectional studies

Table 7-1. Critical Analysis Questions

Type of Question:	Therapy/Prevention		Diagnosis	Prognosis	Harm/Etiology/Causation
Type of Study	Meta-analysis (MA) or Systematic Review (SR) of RCTs, Single RCT SR of Cohort Studies Single Cohort Study	RCTs are needed to evaluate cause & effect. Experimental design allows for randomization of subjects, intervention & double-blinding to minimize bias.	MA or SR of Controlled Trials, Single Controlled Trial Prospective Cohort Study	MA or SR of Inception Cohort Studies, Individual Inception Cohort Study, Cohort Study	MA or SR of Cohort Studies Single Cohort Study Case Controlled Study
KEY QUESTIONS Are the Results of the Study (trial) Valid?	Did the trial or review address a clearly focused question?	If the trial is too broad it may not provide an accurate picture of the therapy.	Were the right patients enrolled in the study and were representative of those with the clinical problem?	Was there a defined, representative sample of patients assembled at a common (usually early) point in the course of their disease and free of the outcome of interest?	Were there clearly defined groups of patients, similar in all important ways other than exposure to the treatment or other cause?
	Is a trial (RCT) an appropriate method to answer this issue? Did the review include the appropriate type of studies?	The study design should match the methodology to demonstrate cause and effect.	Was there a clearly identified comparison group, at least one of which was free from the target disorder?	Were the patients sufficiently similar in regards to prognostic risk?	Were treatments/exposures and clinical outcomes measured in the same ways in the groups being compared (was the assessment of outcomes either objective or blinded to exposure)?
	How were patients assigned to treatment groups? *Did reviewers identify all relevant studies?*	This method should be rigorous to eliminate potential bias.	Was there an independent, blind comparison with a reference ("gold") standard of diagnosis?	Was there follow-up of at least 80% of the patient until the occurrence of either a major study endpoint or end of the study?	Was the follow-up of study patients sufficiently complete?
Is it worth continuing?	Were participants, staff and study personnel 'blind' to groups and treatment? *Did reviewers assess the quality of included studies?*	Again, the data collection & treatment allocation should reflect rigorous methods to maintain quality & minimize bias.	Was the reference standard applied regardless of the diagnostic test result? Was the diagnostic process credible?	Were objective and unbiased outcome criteria applied in a "blind" fashion?	Do the results satisfy some "diagnostic tests for causation"? • Is it clear that the exposure preceded the onset of the outcome? • Is there a dose-response gradient? • Is there positive evidence from a "dechallenge-rechallenge" study? • Is the association consistent from study to study?

Table 7-1. Critical Analysis Questions (continued)

	Therapy/Prevention		Diagnosis	Prognosis	Harm/Etiology/Causation
Is it worth continuing?	Were all the participants who entered the trial properly accounted for at its conclusion? *If the results of the studies were combined, was it reasonable to do so?*	Participants that do not complete the study can skew the SR-results & for the SR-data should compare apples to apples and oranges to oranges.	For initially undiagnosed patients, was follow-up sufficiently long and complete?	If subgroups with different prognoses are identified, was there adjustment for important prognostic factors?	Does the association make biological sense?
	Aside from the experimental intervention, were the groups treated in the same way?	The elimination of additional variables provides a more accurate result.	Was the test (or cluster of tests) validated in a second, independent group of patients?	Was there validation in an independent group ("test set") of patients?	Did both groups retain a similar prognosis after the start of the study?
	Did the study have enough participants to minimize the play of chance?	Sample size is important. Validity is increased with larger sample sizes.			
What are the Results? **Is it worth continuing?**	How are the results presented? What is the main result?	Results should be presented in appropriate measurements and values for the methods.	What were the diagnoses and their probabilities?	Over time, how likely are the outcomes?	How strong is the association between outcome and exposure?
	How precise are these results? [p values & confidence intervals]	The values should show statistical significance. Are the values also clinically relevant?	How precise are the estimates of disease probability?	How precise are the estimates of likelihood?	How precise is the estimate of risk?
Will the results help in caring for my patient?	Can the results be applied to my patient?**	Likelihood of attaining the same results may increase when the study population closely resembles your patient	These questions also will be covered in Chapter 8.	These questions also will be covered in Chapter 8.	These questions also will be covered in Chapter 8.
	Were all important outcomes considered?	Valuable to look at outcomes that reflect the patients' culture, values and beliefs.			

Adapted from CASP Appraisal Tools: http://www.casp-uk.net/casp-tools-checklists and the Users' Guides to the Medical Literature, therapy or prevention A, http://jama.jamanetwork.com/article.aspx?articleid=409494 and B, http://jama.jamanetwork.com/article.aspx?articleid=361625

For a patient with **burning mouth syndrome**, will **tricyclic anti-depressants**, as compared to **benzodiazepines**, be more effective in **relieving the burning sensation on his lips and tongue**?

The highest level of evidence found is the Systematic Review by Zakrzewska J and Buchanan JA, "Burning Mouth Syndrome."[3] This SR categorized the efficacy for six interventions, two of which were tricyclic anti-depressants and benzodiazepines from the PICO question. This SR is an update of an earlier review, adding 10 new studies.

Even though a SR represents synthesized studies that investigate the same question, it is necessary to review the evidence to determine if the methods were conducted rigorously and appropriately. The strength of the evidence derived from the SR depends on the quality of the previously published original studies.

The CASP SR form was used to evaluate the credibility of the SR. A completed form is found in Figure 7-1.

Another facet of reporting should include the source of funding. For example, this could be grant funding from federal agencies, professional associations or contracts from private industry. Again, researchers will want to thoroughly report each aspect of their study to demonstrate how bias is minimized or eliminated.

In addition to the criteria for reporting RCTs and SRs/MAs, there are the Standards for Reporting of Diagnostic Accuracy (STARD), and STrengthening the Reporting of OBservational studies in Epidemiology (STROBE). Both of these can be found at www.equator-network.org. Again, the criteria are designed to improve the reporting of a study, which also helps readers judge the potential for bias in the study and to appraise the applicability of the findings.

The second key question, "What are the results?" refers to the outcomes being considered. They may be reported as yes/no, e.g., caries/caries-free, or using more involved statistical analysis. Results may be presented in terms or risk reduction, odds ratios and numbers needed to treat. These will be more fully explained in Chapter 8.

Once the study is thought to be valid, the final key question, "Will the results help in caring for my patient?" can be determined by asking, "Would my patient have qualified to be in the study?" If yes, then the evidence should be incorporated into the decision making process. However, this may not be the situation in all cases. There could be age, ethnicity, or level of disease differences between those subjects in the study and your patient to the degree that the evidence may not be relevant or cannot be extrapolated to your patient. In these situations, the decision making process will only take into account the practitioner's experience and judgment along with the patient's clinical condition and preferences, the other three components of EBDM.

CONCLUSION

This chapter outlined the third skill in the EBDM process, critical appraisal of the evidence to determine its validity and relevance to the patient problem. In order to successfully complete this step, it is important to understand research design and how the different methodologies relate to the questions being asked. To assist with the process, evidence-based groups have developed tools to critically appraise a range of different study designs. These tools consist of a structured series of questions that help determine the validity by exploring the strengths and weaknesses of how a study was conducted, or of how information was collected, and how useful and applicable the evidence is to the specific patient problem or question being asked.

Figure 7-1. 10 questions to help you make sense of a review

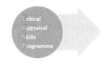

These questions are designed to help you think about these issues systematically. The first two questions are screening questions and can be answered quickly. If the answer to both is "yes", it is worth proceeding with the remaining questions. There is some degree of overlap between the questions, you are asked to record a "yes", "no" or "can't tell" to most of the questions. A number of prompts are given after each question. These are designed to remind you why the question is important. Record your reasons for your answers in the spaces provided.

(A) Are the results of the review valid?

Screening Questions

1. Did the review address a clearly focused question? ☑ Yes _____ Can't tell _____ No

HINT: An issue can be 'focused' In terms of
- The population studied
- The intervention given
- The outcome considered

2. Did the authors look for the right type of papers? ☑ Yes _____ Can't tell _____ No

HINT: 'The best sort of studies' would
- Address the reviews question
- Have an appropriate study design
  (usually RCTs for papers evaluating interventions)

☐ searched for evidence from RCTs and systematic reviews of RCTs on selected interventions in people with burning mouth syndrome

Is it worth continuing?

3. Do you think all the important, relevant studies were included? _____ Yes ☑ Can't tell _____ No

HINT - Look for: Which bibliographic databases were used

- Follow up from reference lists
- Personal contact with experts
- Search for unpublished & published studies
- Search for non-English language studies

☐ Medline 1966 to January 2015, Embase 1980 to January 2015, The Cochrane Database of Systematic Reviews 2015, issue 1 (1966 to date of issue), the Database of Abstracts of Reviews of Effects (DARE), and the Health Technology Assessment (HTA) database.

☐ Unclear

☐ evidence team, editorial team, and expert contributors

☐ Unclear

☐ No

4. Did the review's authors do enough to assess the quality of the included studies? ☑ Yes _____ Can't tell _____ No

HINT: The authors need to consider the rigour of the studies they have identified. Lack of rigour may affect the studies' results.

5. If the results of the review have been combined, was it reasonable to do so? _____ Yes _____ Can't tell _____ No

HINT- Consider whether:
- The results were similar from study to study
- The results of all the included studies are clearly displayed
- The results of the different studies are similar
- The reasons for any variations in results are discussed

☐ Results were not combined, "Outcome measures are varied and, even if the same ones are used, they are applied differently, making comparisons of trials difficult."

(B) What are the results?

6. What are the overall results of the review?

HINT- Consider:
- If you are clear about the review's 'bottom line' results
- What these are (numerically if appropriate)
- How were the results expressed (NNT, odds ratio etc)

Categorized the efficacy for six interventions based on information about the effectiveness and safety of
alphalipoic acid- no more efficacious than placebo-need more studies
benzodiazepines – may help but increased dependence over time
cognitive behavioural therapy (CBT) – may help-insufficient evidence
selective serotonin re-uptake inhibitors (SSRIs) - insufficient evidence
tricyclic antidepressants - insufficient evidence- may impact quality of life
benzydamine hydrochloride - insufficient evidence

7. How precise are the results?

HINT: Look at the confidence intervals, if given

☐ No confidence intervals- each intervention graded evidence quality

(C) Will the results help locally?

8. Can the results be applied to the local population? ☑ Yes _____ Can't tell _____ No

HINT - Consider whether: The patients covered by the review could be sufficiently different to your population to cause concern
Your local setting is likely to differ much from that of the review

9. Were all important outcomes considered? ☑ Yes _____ Can't tell _____ No

HINT - Consider: Is there other information you would like to have seen?

10. Are the benefits worth the harms and costs? ☑ Yes _____ Can't tell _____ No

HINT - Consider: Even if this is not addressed by the review, what do you think

☐ Depends on intervention selected

Chapter 7 Assignments - Appraising the Scientific Literature

1. **Complete the following Exercises – see following pages**
   - Exercise 1. Interpreting Abstracts

2. **Answer the following Critical Thinking Questions:**
   a. Discuss the value of answering key appraisal questions.
   b. Explain the difference between validity and reliability.
   c. Compare and contrast the CASP critical appraisal form with the CONSORT and PRISMA forms.
   d. Explain how critical appraisal guidelines improve the quality of research.

3. **Answer the following Self-Reflection Questions:**
   a. What was the one most useful thing you learned in this chapter?
   b. List 2 ways you think you have developed or grown as a result of this chapter?
   c. What problems did you encounter in this chapter, and what if anything, still needs further clarification?
   d. What assignment of this chapter was most helpful in learning critical appraisal and understanding the value of guidelines for different research designs?

Exercise 1 - Interpreting Abstracts

Name:_____ Date:_____

For each of the following abstracts, identify the type of question and study and the critical analysis evaluation tool that should be used.

a. CONSORT   b. PRISMA   c. STARD   d. STROBE

1. ABSTRACT

DATA SOURCES: PubMed, Web of Science and the Cochrane Oral Health Group Trials Register, www.clinicaltrials.gov, www.centerwatch.com and www.clinicalconnection.com databases. Manual searches of a number of dental journals and the reference lists of identified studies were undertaken.

STUDY SELECTION: Human clinical studies comparing implant failure rates in diabetic and non-diabetic patients were considered. Three reviewers independently selected studies.

DATA EXTRACTION AND SYNTHESIS: The definition of implant failure used was complete loss of the implant. Study quality was assessed using the Cochrane risk of bias approach. A narrative summary of the studies and meta-analysis are presented.

RESULTS: Fourteen studies were included (one randomised controlled trial, six controlled clinical trials and seven retrospective analysis); all 14 were considered to be at high risk of bias. Meta-analysis (14 studies) found no significant difference between diabetic and non-diabetic patients; risk ratio of 1.07 (95% CI = 0.80, 1.44)(p = 65). A meta-analysis of two studies found a statistically significant difference (mean difference =0.20, 95% CI = 0.08, 0.31 p = 001;) between diabetic and non-diabetic patients concerning marginal bone loss, favouring non-diabetic patients. Meta-analysis was not possible for postoperative infections.

CONCLUSIONS: The results of the present systematic review should be interpreted with caution because of the presence of uncontrolled confounding factors in the included studies. Within the limits of the existing investigations, the difference between the insertion of dental implants in non-diabetic and diabetic patients did not statistically affect the implant failure rates.

Type of Question_____ Type of Study_____ Appraisal Guideline_____

2. ABSTRACT

OBJECTIVE: The disease specific five-year survival rate especially for patients with advanced oral cancer has not improved significantly over the period of time. The most effective way of combating this dilemma is an early detection, diagnosis and eradication of early-stage lesions and their precursors. The use of VELscope® using an autofluorescence as a diagnostic tool might be useful in early detection of oral malignant lesions.

MATERIALS AND METHODS: 120 patients with suspicious oral premalignant lesions were examined with two examination methods. They were randomly divided into two groups. Group 1 was examined conventional with white-light and group 2 was examined additionally to the white-light-examination with an autofluorescence visualization device, VELscope®. Biopsies were obtained from all suspicious areas identified in both examination groups (n = 52). The diagnostic strategies were compared regarding sensitivity and specificity.

RESULTS: Based upon the result, use of the VELscope® leads to a higher sensitivity (22.0%), but regarding specificity the additional use of the VELscope® is inferior (8.4%).

CONCLUSION: The VELscope device is a simple, non-invasive test of the oral mucosa, which can help the experienced clinician to find oral precursor malignant lesions.

Type of Question_____ Type of Study_____ Appraisal Guideline_____

For each of the following abstracts, identify the type of question and study and the critical analysis evaluation tool that should be used.

a. CONSORT   b. PRISMA   c. STARD   d. STROBE

3. ABSTRACT

OBJECTIVES: Maintaining good oral hygiene is important to combat periodontal diseases. The use of tooth brush alone does not serve the purpose, especially in inaccessible areas like proximal embrasures, which demand the use of some adjuncts like proximal cleaning aids. Hence, the objective of this study was to compare the clinical efficacy of two antimicrobial mouth rinses (Cool mint Listerine and 0.2% Chlorhexidine gluconate) with dental floss in reducing interproximal gingivitis and dental plaque in an unsupervised condition.

MATERIALS AND METHODS: A randomized, controlled, single-blind (observer), parallel-group clinical trial in accordance with the ADA guidelines was conducted for a period of 6 months. Four index age groups (12, 15, 35-44, and 65-74 years) were divided into four groups, i.e., brushing, brushing and flossing, brushing and rinsing with Listerine, and brushing and rinsing with Chlorhexidine, so that each group comprised 40 subjects. Interproximal gingivitis and dental plaque were assessed using Modified Gingival Index, Turesky-Gilmore-Glickman modified Quigley-Hein Plaque Index and Gingival Bleeding Index. Analysis of variance (ANOVA) was used for multiple group comparisons, followed by Tukey's post hoc for group-wise comparisons.

RESULTS: Chlorhexidine and Listerine showed significant reduction in plaque and gingivitis level compared to others, the activity of Chlorhexidine being more significant.

CONCLUSIONS: The level of interproximal gingivitis control efficacy provided by the Listerine and Chlorhexidine was "at least as good as" that provided by the dental floss. Hence, they can be recommended for the patients with gingivitis as an adjunctive to the usual home care routine.

Type of Question_____   Type of Study_____   Appraisal Guideline_____

4. ABSTRACT

OBJECTIVE: The purpose of this study was to examine the effects of various product combinations involving brush, paste, rinse, and floss on the prevention of plaque regrowth and gingivitis.

METHODOLOGY: In this randomized, parallel-group, examiner-blind, eight-week study, 179 subjects with gingivitis had a dental prophylaxis and were randomly assigned to one of six product combinations: 1) Colgate Wave manual toothbrush + Colgate Total dentifrice (0.3% triclosan/copolymer dentifrice); 2) Wave + Total + Listerine (essential oils rinse); 3) Oral-B CrossAction manual toothbrush + Crest Pro-Health dentifrice (0.454% stannous fluoride/sodium hexametaphosphate); 4) CrossAction + Pro-Health dentifrice + Crest Pro-Health Rinse (0.07% cetylpyridinium chloride rinse); 5) Oral-B ProfessionalCare Series 8000 power toothbrush + Pro-Health dentifrice; or 6) ProfessionalCare power brush + Pro-Health dentifrice + Oral-B Hummingbird power flosser. Subjects used their test products for the duration of the study. Whole mouth plaque, gingivitis, and product-related adverse events were assessed. Treatments were compared at a 0.05 level of significance.

RESULTS: One-hundred and seventy-four subjects completed the study and were included in the data analysis. At Week 8, the overnight adjusted whole mouth plaque scores were statistically significantly lower in all other groups relative to the Wave + Total group (p < or = 0.030). Plaque scores were also statistically significantly lower (approximately 20%) in both groups where a therapeutic rinse was added to a manual brush and therapeutic paste relative to scores for the brush plus paste without a rinse (p < or = 0.034). All groups showed a reduction in gingivitis at Week 4, and mean scores remained stable or increased slightly at Week 8. The power toothbrush groups were directionally better at preventing gingivitis than the manual groups at Weeks 4 and 8.

CONCLUSION: Reductions in overnight plaque were seen when therapeutic rinses were added to manual brush plus therapeutic dentifrice regimens above that observed with a manual brush and therapeutic dentifrice alone.

Type of Question_____   Type of Study_____   Appraisal Guideline_____

References

1.   Greenhalgh T. Getting your bearings (deciding what the paper is about), BMJ 1997; July 26;315 (7102):243-6.

2.   Guyatt G, Rennie D, Meade MO, Cook DJ editors. User's Guide to the Medical Literature, A Manual for Evidence-Based Clinical Practice, 3rd Ed. JAMAevidence, JAMA, Chicago: McGraw Hill Medical, 2015.

3.   Zakrzewska J, Buchanan JA. Burning mouth syndrome. BMJ Clin Evid. 2016 Jan 7; 2016. pii: 1301.

NOTES

CHAPTER

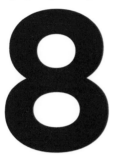

8

APPLYING THE RESULTS

Learning Objectives:
Upon completion of this chapter readers will be able to
1. Discuss how presentation of statistics can influence treatment decisions
2. Identify the differences between absolute and relative risk
3. Distinguish between statistical and clinical significance
4. Identify techniques that can increase the likelihood of obtaining statistical significance
5. Discuss clinical significance in terms of benefits and effect
6. Given a forest plot, statistical significance and outcome of meta-analysis
7. Apply evidence to patients

The purpose of this section is to discuss the fourth step in the EBDM process, applying the results of the evidence into clinical practice. This step involves understanding the type of statistical analysis needed to determine if the valid results found are important and, if so, are they reasonable to implement with the specific patient.   Understanding how to present statistical information to patients in a clear and unambiguous manner will help in making good patient care decisions. In addition, understanding the clinical significance of research findings and translation of the findings to the individual patient is an important aspect of the fourth step.

DDS/DMD CODA STANDARDS
EDUCATIONAL ENVIRONMENT, Critical Thinking:
The components of critical thinking are: the application of logic and accepted intellectual standards to reasoning; the ability to access and evaluate evidence; the application of knowledge in clinical reasoning; and a disposition for inquiry that includes openness, self-assessment, curiosity, skepticism, and dialogue. Students must be able to... Interpret information accurately and arrive at well-reasoned conclusions

EDUCATIONAL ENVIRONMENT, Evidence-based Care:
Evidence-based dentistry (EBD) is an approach to oral health care that requires the judicious integration of systematic assessments of clinically relevant scientific evidence, relating to the patient's oral and medical condition and history, with the dentist's clinical expertise and the patient's treatment needs and preferences.

Clinical Sciences, 2-22 Graduates must be competent to access, critically appraise, apply, and communicate scientific and lay literature as it relates to providing evidence-based patient care.

Patient Care Services, 5-2 Patient care must be evidenced-based, integrating the best research evidence and patient values.

DH CODA STANDARDS
Patient Care Competencies, 2-13 Graduates must be competent in providing the dental hygiene process of care which includes: d) provision of patient-centered treatment and evidence-based care in a manner minimizing risk and optimizing oral health.

Critical Thinking, 2-23: Graduates must be competent in problem solving strategies related to comprehensive patient care and management of patients.

"FACTS ON STATS"

ABSOLUTE AND RELATIVE DIFFERENCES

When applying results of evidence to patient care decisions it is important to understand what the numbers mean so that the information and risks can be communicated in a manner that the patient can understand. This involves explaining the risk of treatment vs. no treatment or a comparison treatment. This is considered crucial for appropriate decision-making, and yet this can be very challenging.[1] Two of the most common ways risk/benefit information is presented is through the use of absolute and relative terms.[2]

- **Absolute risk or absolute risk ratio (ARR)** is the arithmetic difference between two rates, i.e., an event occurring in an exposed group minus the event occurring in a comparison, non-exposed group (A-B).
- **Relative risk or risk ratio (RR)** is the ratio of the probability of an event occurring (e.g., developing a disease, being injured) in an exposed group to the probability of the event occurring in a comparison, non-exposed group, i.e., a ratio (B/A).

To illustrate the difference, consider a hypothetical case looking at the risk of implant failure after 5 years. If the risk is 6 in 100 (6%) for those treated using implant A, and 3 in 100 (3%) for those treated using implant B, the **absolute difference** is calculated by subtracting, 6% - 3% = 3%. This can be stated as implant B reduces the risk of implant failure by 3%. The **relative risk difference** is the ratio of the 2 risks, 3% ÷ 6% = ½ or 50% and can be state as implant B reduces the risk of implant failure by 50%.

Based on the presentation of the results in absolute terms (3% reduction) or in relative terms (50% reduction), clinicians could decide to start using implant B or stop using it thinking that 3% difference (3 patients) is too small to change from using implant A to implant B. Factored into this decision would be the time, cost, number of patients actually needing implants, and number of visits required to determine if the outcome is worthwhile. Not surprisingly, investigators have found that clinicians judge a therapy to be less effective when the results are presented in absolute terms,[3,4] which parallels the finding that patients are more likely to select a treatment when described in terms of relative risk reduction.[5,6]

The problem with reporting the relative risk/benefits in the literature is that the starting or reference point is not typically given. Using our example of reducing implant failure, the report may just say that there is a 50% reduction in implant failure when using implant B. The starting point of 6 of 100 patients is not given so that reducing the risk of failure by half or 50% refers now only to 3 patients having implants that do not fail.

Another, and perhaps a simpler and easier to understand description of the same information is using frequency rates. For example, for every 100 patients who have an implant placed, 6 will fail using implant A and 3 will fail using implant B after a 5-year period. This presentation talks about a negative outcome. Another way to present the same information is to present the

---

ARR vs. RR

RISK OF IMPLANT
FAILURE IN 5 YEARS

Presentation of results can influence decison-making.

Implant A: 6 patients out of 100 fail

Implant B: 3 patients out of 100 fail

AAR= 6% - 3% = 3%

RR = $\frac{3\%}{6\%}$ or $\frac{1}{2}$ or **50%**

The same results can represent a very different message.

information in terms of a positive outcome, that is for every 100 patient, 94 will survive more than 5 years using implant A, whereas 97 will survive using implant B. These scenarios demonstrate the difference between negative and positive verbal framing, which can influence the perceptions of the risk or benefit and how decisions are made.[1,7] Even though the information may be correct, presenting outcomes using relative findings rather than absolute differences tend to inflate the size of the effect.

STATISTICAL & CONFIDENCE INTERVAL (CI)

Statistics is the study of the collection, analysis, interpretation, presentation and organization of data so that they can be communicated in a meaningful way.[8] In most cases, measurements cannot be taken on everyone in the population, so a random, representative sample of the population is selected, which helps assure that inferences and conclusions can safely extend from the sample back to the population as a whole. **A statistic is a characteristic of a sample**, such as an average or mean.

Statistics involve proposing a hypothesis and testing the relationship between sets of data, e.g., mouthwash A will decrease gingivitis more effectively than mouthwash B. This is compared to a null hypothesis, which states there is no relationship or no difference between the data sets, i.e., no difference between mouthwash A and mouthwash B in their effectiveness to decrease gingivitis.

Statistical significance refers to the likelihood that an intervention had an effect, i.e., the results did not occur by chance at a pre-specified probability level and that the differences would still exist each time the experiment was repeated. Therefore, statistical significance is reported as the **probability related to chance, or "p" level**. Levels of statistical significance are set at thresholds (the cut off level for determining significance), which is the point where the null hypothesis (the statement of no difference between groups) will be rejected. Often the threshold is set at $p < 0.05$, where the probability is less than 5 in 100, or 1 in 20 that the difference occurred by chance. Using the mouthwash example, after comparing the two mouthwashes, the resulting "p" level was $p < 0.03$ (where the probability is less than 3 in 100 that the difference occurred by chance). Since this meets the threshold set at $p < 0.05$, the **null hypothesis would be rejected indicating that there was a significant difference between the two mouthwashes in decreasing gingivitis**. This could be stated as, there is a statistically significant difference between mouthwash A and mouthwash B, and mouthwash A is more effective than mouthwash B in decreasing gingivitis.

If the threshold had been set at $p < 0.01$ (less than 1 in 100 that the difference occurred by chance), and the resulting analysis of $p < 0.03$ would not have met the threshold. In this case, the null hypothesis would not be rejected. This result would be stated as there is no statistically significant difference between mouthwash A and mouthwash B in decreasing gingivitis.

STATISTICS

1. The study of the
   • collection
   • analysis
   • interpretation and
   • organization
of data so that they can be communicated in a meaningful way.

2. involve proposing a hypothesis and testing the relationship between sets of data.

NULL HYPOTHESIS

1. states there is no difference between data sets

2. when a statistically significant difference is found, the null hypothesis is rejected

CONFIDENCE INTERVAL

A range of values that describes the uncertainty surrounding an estimate or how well the sample mean estimates the mean of the population it was taken from.

Expectation that the true population parameter will fall within the interval estimate 95% of the time.

In a study comparing two different placement techniques for sealants, the mean difference in sealant loss in the two groups was 8 with a 95% CI of ± 2 sealants. This means that if the study was repeated 100 times, the mean difference in sealant loss would be between 6 and 10 sealants (8 ± 2) for 95% of the trials.[9]

Another concept related to statistical significance is the **Confidence Interval** (CI), which quantifies the precision or uncertainty associated with the sample statistic, or how well the sample mean estimates the mean of the population from which it was taken. The CI addresses this by providing a range of values, which is likely to contain the population mean. The CI usually is reported as 95% CI, which is the range of values within which we can be 95% sure that the true value for the whole population lies.[9] So, if we used the same sampling method to select different samples from the same population and computed an interval estimate for each sample, we would expect the true population parameter to fall within the interval estimates 95% of the time.[9] For example, in a study comparing two different placement techniques for sealants, the mean difference in sealant loss in the two groups was 8 with a 95% CI of ± 2 sealants. This means that if the study was repeated 100 times, the mean difference in sealant loss would be between 6 and 10 sealants (8 ± 2) for 95% of the trials.[9]

Statistical significance does not determine the practical or clinical significance of the data. For example, in a comparison study of 2 treatments to relieve hyposalivation after radiation therapy, a salivary flow rate increase of 3 mg/5 minutes may be statistically significant, however this increase may not be clinically significant in helping to relieve a patient's dry mouth. Conversely, the increase in flow rate may not be statistically significant, and yet patients may report that it made a difference suggesting that even minor increases in saliva may produce a clinical significant and quality of life benefit.[10]

Be mindful in interpreting results and their implications. Just because there is no statistically significant difference between two treatments or between two diagnostic tests, does not mean that the finding is not important. For example, the investigation could be determining if a new treatment or diagnostic test is as effective as the current gold standard. In this case, if there is no significant difference between the two treatments or two diagnostic tests it could mean the new treatment or new diagnostic test is as effective as the gold standard.

Statistical significance is an important tool for determining the validity of a study's results, however a number of techniques can increase the likelihood of obtaining statistically significant results. For example, as a **sample size increases**, the group differences needed to reach the "p" level decreases. Therefore, any difference between treatment groups can become statistically significant if the studies are conducted with large enough sample sizes, however this does not mean they are clinically important. Also, **decreasing the variability within groups** is another technique that will increase the likelihood that the differences between groups will be significant.[11] Thus, statistically significant results can be incomplete and provide misleading conclusions.[11]

CLINICAL SIGNIFICANCE

Clinical significance is used to distinguish the importance and meaning of the results reported in a study and is **not based on a comparison of numbers**, as is statistical significance. It is possible for a study to have statistical significance without being clinically significant and vice versa. Statistical significance does not determine the practical or clinical implications of the data. For example, a new periodontal treatment "x" may increase levels of attachment .05 to 1.0 mm more than the standard treatment "y", which may be statistically significant; however, this small a difference may not be clinically important in terms of saving periodontally compromised teeth. Also, the new treatment "x" provided to obtain these results may not take into account any additional training, special materials, new instruments, patient time and/or cost.

Hujoel discusses clinical significance in terms of **tangible versus intangible benefits**, defining tangible as "those treatment outcomes that reflect how a patient feels, functions or survives."[12,p.32]   These benefits include those that **can be identified by the patient**, such as improving quality of life, prevention of tooth loss or eliminating a painful abscess. On the other hand, **intangible benefits** are imperceptible to the patient and include such changes in probing depths due to scaling, the size of a periapical radiolucency after root canal treatment, or the reduction in bacteria after using an antiseptic rinse. [12] Hujoel also points out that intangible benefits do not neatly translate into tangible benefits, even though a clinician can often measure them. Consequently, a treatment that provides tangible benefits has a higher level of clinical significance. Ideally, clinical significant treatments also would have intangible benefits.[12]

Another criterion for assessing clinical significance is the size of the **treatment effect**, i.e., a comparison of the success rates of the experimental and the control treatment. For treatments that achieve a dramatic and immediate effect, reliable evidence may result from observations on a small number of patients, e.g., the effectiveness of general anesthesia. In contrast, for small treatment effects, large, rigorously designed controlled trials are required. The more likely a patient's preferences and tangible benefits are achieved, the greater the clinical significance of the treatment.[12]

In a meta-analysis, the effect size is a measure of the difference between two groups, calculated based on the standardized mean difference (SMD), i.e., the difference between the average score of participants in the intervention group and the the average score of those in the control group. Unlike statistical significance where all studies are treated equally, in a meta-analysis, the effect size takes into account the sample size and gives more weight to a study with more participants.[13] Also, by synthesizing the results and pooling the data from the individual studies, an overall summary estimate can be calculated. Results can either confirm or strengthen the findings from smaller studies, or find that treatments may not be as effective as originally thought.

FOREST PLOTS

Results of a meta-analysis are typically displayed in a **forest plot**, as seen in Figure 8-1.[14] Forest plots display the relative strength of treatment effects from multiple individual studies that address the same question. They show the between study spread of

---

TANGIBLE BENEFITS[12]

Treatment outcomes that reflect how a patient feels, functions or survives

- Improving quality of life
- prevention of tooth loss
- eliminating pain

INTANGIBLE BENEFITS[12]

Treatment outcomes Imperceptible to patient

- probing depth
- periapical radiolucency
- reduction in bacteria

results from all the studies combined. As presented on the Centre for Evidence-Based Medicine's (CEBM's) Systematic Review Critical Appraisal Worksheet (cebm.net/critical-appraisal). Under "How are the results presented?" the meta-analysis gives weighted values to each of the individual studies according to their size.[13] In this case, the odds ratio (OR) is used to express the results in a standard way.

ODDS RATIOS (OR)

The proportion of patients with the target event divided by the proportion of patients without the event. Odds Ratios often are used to report results when data from several studies are combined since the OR is not dependent on whether the risk of an event occurring was determined.

Figure 8-1. A Forest Plot[14]
Permission to reproduce the forest plot granted by the Centre for Evidence-Based Medicine's Systematic Review Critical Appraisal Worksheet, English, (http://www.cebm.net/critical-appraisal/)

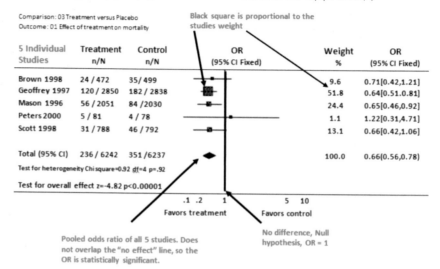

The forest plot depicted represents a meta-analysis of 5 trials that assessed the effects of a hypothetical treatment on mortality. Individual studies are represented by a black square. The horizontal line going through the square represents the confidence interval. These correspond to the point estimate (mean) and 95% confidence interval of the odds ratio.[14]

The size of the black square is proportional to the study's weight in the meta-analysis. As you can see on the forest plot, the first study by Brown had the second fewest participants and therefore the black square is proportionately smaller as is the weighted percent than larger studies. In comparison, the second study by Geoffrey had the largest number of participants and accounts for the largest weighted percent.

The solid vertical line corresponds to the null hypothesis or 'no effect' of treatment - an odds ratio of 1.0. When the confidence interval includes 1 (touches or crosses the line) it indicates that the result is not significant at conventional levels (P>0.05). The diamond at the bottom represents the combined or pooled odds ratio of all 5 trials with its 95% confidence interval. In this case, it shows that the treatment reduces mortality by 34% (OR 0.66, 95% CI 0.56, 0.78). Since the diamond does not overlap the 'no effect' line (the confidence interval doesn't include 1) the pooled OR is statistically significant. The test for overall effect also indicates statistical significance (p<0.0001).[14] **For further information about Forest Plots, check out the youtube video: https://www.youtube.com/watch?v=py-L8DvJmDc**

APPLYING EVIDENCE TO PRACTICE

To determine clinical significance one must go beyond the statistics and use all aspects of the evidence-based decision-making process, i.e., the patient's preferences and values, and the clinical circumstances in combination with the clinician's experience and judgment. Some helpful questions to consider when determining clinical significance are outlined in Table 8-1. Using evidence-based decision making, scientific evidence is only one component to the decision making process. Synthesizing all four components, which are represented in the table, is key to deciding a course of action for your patient.

TABLE 8-1. Questions to ask prior to applying evidence to practice

				Rationale
1. Are the study groups similar enough to apply to my patient?	YES	NO	CAN'T TELL	
2. Is this available, affordable, & appropriate for the patient in this setting?	YES	NO	CAN'T TELL	
3. Will this help the patient meet his/her goals or address their chief complaint?	YES	NO	CAN'T TELL	
4. Is the difference large enough to warrant the treatment?	YES	NO	CAN'T TELL	
5. Are there adverse effects that influence a potential recommendation?	YES	NO	CAN'T TELL	

Summary of Scientific Evidence:	Summary of Your Experience/Judgment:	Summary of Patient Preferences/Values:	Summary of Patient 's Clinical Condition/ Circumstances

Overall Recommendations to the patient based on the EBDM process:

CONCLUSION

After the methods are determined to be valid, the next step is to determine if the results, potential benefits or harms, are important. This is achieved by looking at whether there is an association between specific treatments and outcomes/exposures, and the condition of interest, and then the strength of that association. Differences between groups in clinical trials are generally straight forward when expressed in terms of the mean values; whereas, results presented as proportions, such as relative risk reduction and absolute risk reduction, are more challenging to understand.[1]

Understanding how statistical findings are presented can be difficult, especially since these may not have been part of a clinician's formal education. Even though the information may be correct, presenting outcomes using relative findings rather than absolute differences tend to inflate the size of the effect and can influence a patient to accept the treatment a clinician may want the patient to select. In determining clinical significance, it is important to go beyond the statistics and to consider all components of the decision-making process.

Chapter 8 Assignments - Applying the Results

1. **Complete the following Exercises – see following pages**
   E1: Absolute & Relative Risk
   E2: Forest Plot Identification
   E3: Application of Evidence

2. **Answer the following Critical Thinking Questions:**
   a. Discuss how the presentation of results in absolute or relative terms can influence a decision.

   b. Identify situations when clinical significance will outweigh statistical significance and vice versa.

   c. Describe why it is important that the study sample population groups are similar to your patient.

3. **Answer the following Self-Reflection Questions:**
   a. What was the one most useful thing you learned in this unit?

   b. List 2 ways you think you have developed or grown as a result of this unit?

   c. What did you learn about writing, research, (or an EB skill) from this unit?

   d. What problems did you encounter in this unit, and what if anything, still needs further clarification?

   e. What assignment of this unit was most helpful in learning about applying the results of the appraisal, or evidence, in clinical practice?

Exercise 1 - Absolute and Relative Risk

You have just read a journal article stating that a new preventive product will reduce the 3-year risk of tooth loss for diabetic patients by 60%. However, you are not quite sure what this truly means.

1.   Identify 3 questions you should have answers to so that you more clearly understand what is meant by an 60% reduction?

2.   How can you present the information in terms that your patients will have a clear understanding of what an 60% reduction means?

3.   Present the information using both positive and negative framing.
      a.   Positive:
      b.   Negative

Exercise 2 - Interpreting information from a Forest Plot

Forest Plot

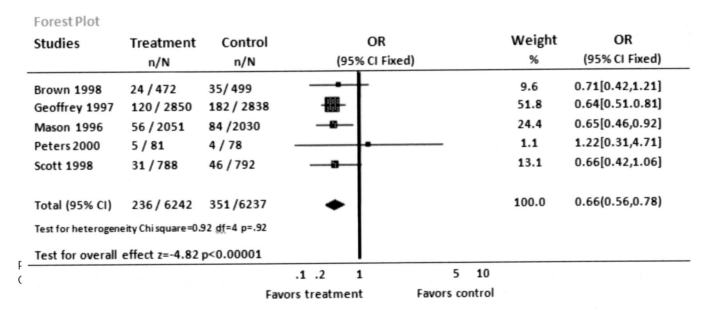

Studies	Treatment n/N	Control n/N	OR (95% CI Fixed)	Weight %	OR (95% CI Fixed)
Brown 1998	24 / 472	35/ 499		9.6	0.71[0.42,1.21]
Geoffrey 1997	120 / 2850	182 / 2838		51.8	0.64[0.51.0.81]
Mason 1996	56 / 2051	84 /2030		24.4	0.65[0.46,0.92]
Peters 2000	5 / 81	4 / 78		1.1	1.22[0.31,4.71]
Scott 1998	31 / 788	46 / 792		13.1	0.66[0.42,1.06]
Total (95% CI)	236 / 6242	351 /6237		100.0	0.66(0.56,0.78)

Test for heterogeneity Chi square=0.92 df=4 p=.92

Test for overall effect z=-4.82 p<0.00001

.1 .2   1   5   10

Favors treatment   Favors control

1.   Identify the study weighted the least and a reason why:

2.   Identify the study weighted the most and a reason why:

3.   Identify all of the studies that are statistically significant and how this was determined:

4.   What is the overall outcome of the meta-analysis and two characteristics/items that support your answer?

Exercise 3 - Applying the Evidence

After reading the article "Burning Mouth Syndrome" by Zakrzewska and Buchanan, answer the following questions to determine the answer to Nathan's PICO question and which, if any, of the treatments you recommend to Nathan.

PICO Question for Nathan: For a patient with BMS, will tricyclic anti-depressants, compared to benzodiazepines, be more effective in relieving the burning sensation on his lips and tongue?

	YES	NO	CAN'T TELL	Rationale
1. Are the study groups similar enough to apply to my patient?	YES	NO	CAN'T TELL	
2. Is this available, affordable, & appropriate for the patient in this setting?	YES	NO	CAN'T TELL	
3. Will this help the patient meet his/her goals or address their chief complaint?	YES	NO	CAN'T TELL	
4. Is the difference large enough to warrant the treatment?	YES	NO	CAN'T TELL	
5. Are there adverse effects that influence a potential recommendation?	YES	NO	CAN'T TELL	

Summary of Scientific Evidence:	Summary of Your Experience/Judgment:	Summary of Patient Preferences/Values:	Summary of Patient 's Clinical Condition/ Circumstances

Overall Recommendations to the patient based on the EBDM process:

References

1.   Gigerenzer G, Edwards A. Simple tools for understanding risks: from innumeracy to insight. BMJ 2003; 327:741-744.

2.   McKibbon A, Wilczynski N. PDQ, (Pretty Darned Quick) Evidence-based principles and practice, 2nd Ed. Connecticut, People's Medical Publishing House, 2009.

3.   Guyatt G, Drummond R, Meade M, Cook D. Evidence-based Medicine Working Group. Users' Guides to the Medical Literature, A Manual for Evidence-Based Clinical Practice. 2nd ed. (JAMA & Archives Journals), Chicago: McGraw Hill Medical, 2008.

4.   Froud R, Underwood M, Carnes D, Eldridge S. Clinicians' perceptions of reporting methods for back pain trials: a qualitative study. Br J Gen Pract. 2012 Mar;62(596):e151-9.

5.   Covey J. A meta-analysis of the effects of presenting treatment benefits in different formats. Med Decision Making 2007; 27(5):638–654.

6.   Timmermans D, Molewijk B, Stiggelbout A, Kievit J. Different formats for communicating surgical risks to patients and the effect on choice of treatment. Patient Educ Couns 2004; 54:255-263.

7.   Edwards AGK, Elwyn GJ, Covey J, Mathews E, Pill R. Presenting risk information: a review of the effects of "framing" and other manipulations on patient outcomes. J Health Commun 2001;6:61-82.

8.   Portnoy LG, Watkins MP. Foundations of Clinical Research: Applications to Practice. Mar 18, 2015. Philadelphia: F.A. Davis Company.

9.   Straus S, Glasziou P, Richardson W, Haynes RB. Evidence-Based Medicine: How to Practice and Teach EBM. 5th ed. China, Elsevier Limited, 2019.

10.   Gorsky M, Epstein J, Parry J, Epstein M, Le N, Silverman S. The efficacy of pilocarpine and bethanechol upon saliva production in cancer patients with hyposalivation following radiation therapy. Oral Surg Oral Med Oral Pathol Oral Radiol Endod 2004; 97:190-195.

11.   Glaros A. Statistical and clinical significance: alternative methods for understanding the importance of research findings. J Irish Dent Assoc 2004; 50(3):128-131.

12.   Hujoel P. Levels of Clinical Significance. J Evid Base Dent Pract 2004; 4:32-36.

13.   Center for Evidence Based Intervention (CEBI), University of Oxford. What is an Effect Size? Accessed 2-29-16, www.cebi.ox.ac.uk/for-practitioners/what-is-good-evidence/what-is-an-effect-size.html

14.   Centre for Evidence-Based Medicine. Systematic Review Critical Appraisal Worksheet, How are the results presented? University of Oxford, 2005. Accessed 3-11-19, http://www.cebm.net/critical-appraisal/

EBDM Process Rubric

SCORE	Formulates a well-built question using the PICO format	Conducts an Efficient Computerized Search	Critically Appraises the Evidence for its Validity and Usefulness	Applies the results of the appraisal, or evidence, in clinical practice	Evaluates The Process And Performance
PROFICIENT (DOES) **4** **Expertly Skilled**	Question is clearly focused, stated in the correct format, and effectively outlines the problem using only relevant descriptor(s), a well-defined intervention, a precise comparison and measurable outcome(s) that clearly addresses the problem or patient. Consistently identifies the correct type of question related to levels of evidence and study methodology.	A well-structured search using multiple databases, is clearly developed, & logically executed using effective techniques. Search skillfully demonstrates use of MeSH or alternate terms, filters, and combining terms to maximize the search and produce relevant results that answer the question. Strategy is clearly defined and easily reproducible.	Publications are accurately selected according to the correct type of clinical question, level of evidence and study methodology. Appraisal clearly and logically answered for appraising validity and relevance. Appraisal skillfully demonstrates an understanding of research design components. Knowledgeable analysis of the publication.	Skillful comprehension of the presentation of statistical results and techniques that affect outcomes. Distinctly interprets the results of a forest plot and determines if the results should be incorporated into clinical decision-making. Effortlessly presents information and risks in a manner that patients can understand.	Self-evaluation is thorough and meaningful. Strengths and weaknesses are clearly delineated. Learning needs are specific and relevant. Strategies to meet those needs are descriptive and measurable.
COMPETENT (SHOWS) **3** **Highly Capable**	Question is adequately focused, stated in the correct format, and effectively outlines the problem using a relevant descriptor(s), a clear intervention, a distinct comparison, and measurable outcome(s) that adequately address the problem or patient. Adequately identifies the correct type of question related to levels of evidence and study methodology.	A well-structured search using multiple databases, is adequately developed using effective techniques. Search utilizes MeSH or alternate terms, filters, and combining terms to maximize the search and produce relevant results that answer the question. Strategy is reproducible.	Publications are adequately selected according to the type of clinical question, level of evidence and study methodology. Appraisal understandably answered for appraising validity and relevance. Appraisal demonstrates a clear understanding of research design components. Skillful analysis of the publication.	Adequate understanding of the presentation of statistical results and the techniques that can affect outcomes. Effectively interprets the results of a forest plot and determines if the results should be incorporated into clinical decision-making. Adequately presents information and risks in a manner that patients can understand.	Self-evaluation is significant to task. Strengths and weaknesses are thorough. Learning needs are focused and understandable. Strategies to meet those needs are measurable.
BEGINNNER (KNOWS HOW) **2** **Requires Practice**	Question has a minor drift in focus and vaguely outlines the problem using general descriptors for the P, I, C & O. Components are too general to support an effective search. Question is not clearly stated in the proper format. Inconsistently identifies the correctly type of question related to levels of evidence and study methodology.	A search using 1-2 databases, is conducted using searching skills. It is unclear if the use of MeSH or alternate terms, filters, and combining terms to maximize the search were used effectively. Strategy is unorganized and not easily reproducible.	Publications selected reflect the type of clinical question, level of evidence and study methodology. Appraisal satisfactorily answered for appraising validity and relevance. Appraisal passably demonstrates understanding of research design components. Ineffective analysis of the publication.	Some difficulty understanding the presentation of statistical results and the techniques that can affect outcomes. Passably interprets the results of a forest plot and determines if the results should be incorporated into clinical decision-making. Struggles to present information and risks in a manner that patients can understand. Some difficulty translating evidence into practice.	Self-evaluation is thoughtful. Strengths and weaknesses are clearly stated. Learning needs are well-defined. Strategies to meet those needs are descriptive and measurable.
VICE (KNOWS) **1** **Just Learning**	Question has a major drift in focus and is missing components and/or is not stated in the proper format. Components do not address problem or are so general as to be unlikely to contribute to a relevant search. Unable to correctly identify type of question related to levels of evidence and study methodology.	A search using at least one database is conducted using searching skills. The search is missing MeSH or alternate terms, filters, and combining terms to maximize the search. Strategy is unclear and not reproducible.	Publications are selected but may not be appropriate to the type of clinical question, level of evidence and study methodology. Appraisal not clearly answered for appraising validity and relevance. Does not understand research and how it is interpreted to answer a clinical question.	Unclear understanding the presentation of statistical results and the techniques that can affect outcomes. Confusing interpretation of the results of a forest plot and how it determines if the results should be incorporated into clinical decision-making. Presents information and risks in a manner that is difficult for patients to understand. Does not translate evidence into practice.	Self-evaluation is completed. Strengths and weaknesses are identified. Learning needs are listed. Strategies to meet those needs are defined.
0	No PICO components or question are evident. No type of question identified.	There is no evidence of a computerized search.	No evidence of an appraisal of the research.	Statistics/Reporting of Results not documented. No application to patient.	No evaluation is completed.

EBDM in Action: Developing Competence in Evidence-Based Practice

Absolute Difference	The arithmetic difference between rates.
Absolute Risk Reduction	The absolute arithmetic difference in the event rates between two groups, e.g., the control group (CER) and the experimental group (EER). The formula for its calculation is [C/(C+D)] - [A/(A+B)] or CER-EER. For example, if 10 per cent of people die in the experimental group and 20 per cent in the control group, the ARR is 10 per cent (20–10 per cent).
Background Question	General knowledge inquiry that asks who, what, where, when, how, or why.
Bias	Systematic deviations from the underlying truth. Something that distorts the real effect in a study. Sources of bias can include selection, allocation, attrition, reporting and recall bias.
Blinding/masking	A strategy for preventing individuals/subjects, investigators, and those assessing outcomes in a study from knowing whether the subject was assigned to the experimental or control group.
Boolean operators	Words used to associate terms in a PubMed/MEDLINE search that limit results of a search by allowing the combination of search terms or concepts. The three Boolean operators are **AND, OR** and **NOT.**
Case control studies	Case control studies are retrospective in that subjects *already have a certain disease or condition* and are compared with a representative group of disease-free persons (controls) from the same population. Observations are made about possible associations between the disease of interest (lung cancer) and one or more hypothesized risk factors (tobacco use).[10]
Case report	A description of a single patient case report. These are observations and do not use a control group with which to compare outcomes.
Case series	Descriptions of a series of patients with a similar situation that report observations and do not use a control group with which to compare outcomes.
CINAHL	The Cumulative Index to Nursing & Allied Health an online database that provides access to journals related to nursing and other allied health fields, including dental hygiene
Clinical Decision Support System (CDSS)	Computerized clinical decision support systems (CDSS) are at the top of the hierarchy of evidence-based information resources. When integrated with an electronic health record, the individual patient's characteristics are automatically linked to the current best evidence that matches his or her specific circumstances.[3]
Clinical Practice Guidelines	Systematically developed statements to assist practitioner and patient decisions about appropriate health care for specific clinical circumstances. Not all procedures have a related practice guideline.
Clinical Significance	Clinical significance is used to distinguish the importance and meaning of the results reported in a study and is not based on a comparison of numbers, as is statistical significance. It is possible for a study to have statistical significance without being clinically significant and vice versa. The importance and meaning of the results reported in a study related to tangible and intangible benefits.

Cohort Study	A study that makes observations about the association between a particular exposure or a risk factor (e.g., tobacco use) and the subsequent development of a disease or condition (e.g., lung cancer). In these studies, subjects do not presently have the condition of interest (lung cancer) and are followed over time to see at what frequency they develop the disease/condition as compared to a control group who is not exposed to the risk factor (tobacco use) under investigation.
Confidence Interval (CI)	Covers the likely range of the true effect. Quantifies the precision or uncertainty of study results. It usually is reported as 95% CI, which is the range of values within which we can be 95% sure that the true value for the whole population lies
Control Event Rate	The proportion of patients in the control group (those who did not receive treatment), who experience the event, i.e., tooth loss. The CER formula is C/(C+D).
Critical Summaries (Also see Synopsis)	A synopsis or critically appraised summary of secondary (or primary) research is a 1-2 page critical summary of the SR/MA, or original research article plus an expert commentary. The commentary includes a critique of the strength and weakness of the methodology **and** of the evidence. The commentary concludes with the practical application of the research to practice along with any concerns or precautions.
Diagnosis Questions	Questions that look for evidence to determine the degree to which a test is reliable and useful; the selection and interpretation of diagnostic methods or tests that establish the power of an intervention to differentiate between those with and without a target condition or disease. (See sensitivity and specificity.)
Double blind RCT	Contains the rigor and methodology of an RCT but in addition is conducted so that neither the patient nor the investigator knows whether the patient is receiving the experimental treatment or the control treatment. knowing whether the subject was assigned to the experimental or control group.
Event Rate	The proportion of patients in a group in whom the event is observed.
Evidence-based Decision-Making	The formalized process and structure for using the skills for identifying, searching for and interpreting the results of clinical research so that the best scientific evidence is considered in conjunction with experience and judgment, patient values, and clinical circumstances when making patient care decisions.
Evidence-based journals	Journals that provide concise and easy-to-read summaries of original and review articles selected from the biomedical literature based on specific inclusion criteria.
Evidence-based Medicine	The integration of best research evidence with our clinical expertise and our patient's unique values and circumstances.
Experimental Event Rate	The proportion of patients in the experimental group (those who received treatment), who experience the event, i.e., tooth loss. The EER formula is A/(A+B).
Experimental studies	Studies in which the researcher controls or manipulates the variables under investigation, such as in testing the effectiveness of a treatment. These studies are the most complex and include randomized controlled trials and controlled clinical trials.
Foreground Question	A specific question that is structured to find a precise answer and phrased to facilitate a computerized search. It should include four parts that identify the patient problem or population (P), intervention (I), comparison (C) and outcome(s) (O), referred to as PICO.

Forest Plot	Displays the relative strength of treatment effects from multiple individual studies that address the same question. They show the between study spread of results and provide a summary estimate of the results from all the studies combined.
Gold Standard Test	The test or measure considered the ultimate or ideal.
Grey Literature	Newsletters, reports, working papers, theses, government documents, bulletins, fact sheets, conference proceedings and other publications not controlled by commercial publishers
Harm, Causation, Etiology questions	Questions that are used to identify causes of a disease or condition including iatrogenic forms and to determine relationships between risk factors, potentially harmful agents, and possible causes of a disease or condition.
Inception cohort studies	Studies where the cohort of subjects is all initially free of the outcome of interest and are followed until the occurrence of either a major study endpoint or end of the study.
Levels of evidence	Hierarchy of research study designs that rank the validity of evidence, allowing the user to put confidence in the results.
Likelihood Ratios	The likelihood of a given test result in a patient with the disorder compared to the likelihood of the same result in a patient without the disorder. A positive likelihood ratio (+LR) is calculated as sensitivity/(1-specificity) or $[a/(a+c)]$ ، $1- [b/(b+d)]$; whereas a negative likelihood ratio (-LR) is calculated as (1-sensitivity)/specificity or $1- [a/(a+c)]$ ، $d/(b+d)$.
Medical Subject Headings (MeSH®)	A controlled vocabulary of biomedical terms to index articles, to catalog books and other holdings, and to facilitate searching within MEDLINE
MEDLINE	The bibliographic database of the National Library of Medicine [NLM]. It contains bibliographic citations and author abstracts that cover the fields of medicine, nursing, dentistry, and veterinary medicine
Meta-analysis	The statistical process commonly used with systematic reviews which involves combining the data from multiple individual studies into one analysis.
Negative Predictive Value	The proportion of people with a negative test who do not have the target disorder = $d/(c + d)$.
Non-experimental studies	Studies in which the researcher does not give a treatment, intervention or provide an exposure, i.e., data is gathered without intervening to control variables. Examples of non-experimental studies include cohort studies, case control studies, case series and case reports.
Numbers Needed to Treat	The number of patients (teeth, surfaces, periodontal pockets) that need to be treated with the experimental treatment or intervention in order to have one additional patient (tooth, surface, periodontal pocket) benefit, or to prevent one adverse outcome. NNT is calculated as 1/ARR.
Odds Ratio	The proportion of patients with the target event divided by the proportion without the event, which yields the odds ratio of: [A/B] / [C/D] or AD/BC.
OVID	An information search platform which includes Ovid Gateway and SilverPlatter allows users to access electronic citations, including journals, books, and databases, with innovative tools to browse, search, retrieve, and analyze critical information

PICO	A systematic process for converting information needs/problems into questions so that they can be answered. A "well-built" question includes four parts that identify the patient problem or population (P), intervention (I), comparison (C) and outcome(s) (O), referred to as PICO.1 (Sackett et al. 1997). (Also see Foreground Question)
p Level	Statistical significance is reported as the *probability related to chance, or "p" level.* A threshold for determining significance where the null hypothesis will be rejected.
Placebo	An inert treatment, substance or procedure, one that is not expected to have any effect.
Positive Predictive Value	The proportion of people with a positive test who actually have the target disorder = a/(a + b) or true positives/ (true positives + true negatives).
Primary research	Original research publications that have not been filtered or synthesized and include individual RCTs, and well-designed non-randomized control studies.
Prognosis Questions	Questions that look to studies that estimate the clinical course or progression of a disease or condition over time and anticipate likely complications (and prevent them).
PubMed	An online database that provides free access to citations from biomedical literature, including MEDLINE as well as access and links to other molecular biology resources
Qualitative Research	Non-experimental research that conducts studies in natural settings in an attempt to understand an event from the point of view of the participants. It seeks to provide depth of understanding and does so through answering questions such as what, how and why. It explores issues in more depth with those experiencing the issue rather than testing a hypothesis to answer questions such as how many or what proportion. It uses an interpretive, naturalistic approach that focuses on how individuals or groups view and understand their surroundings and construct meaning out of their experiences.
Quantitative Research	Research that focuses on establishing cause and effect relationships through testing a specific hypothesis and reporting the results in statistical terms.
Randomized-Controlled Trial	Involves at least 1 test/experimental treatment or intervention, and 1 control treatment, which can be a placebo treatment or no treatment. - Concurrent enrollment of subjects and follow-up of the experimental test- and control-treated groups, - Assignment of subjects to either the experimental treatment/intervention group or the control/placebo group through a random process, such as the use of a random-numbers table, and - Follow-up of both groups to determine the outcome.
Recall Bias	A systematic error caused by differences in the completeness of the recollection retrieved by study participants regarding events or experiences from the past, e.g., the number of x-rays an older adult had taken as a teenager.
Relative Risk	Likelihood that someone exposed to a risk factor (or treatment) will develop the disease (or experience a benefit) as compared to one who has not been exposed. The formula is the risk of the event in the exposed or experimental group, **EER** [A/(A+B)] divided by the risk of the event in the unexposed group, **CER** [C/(C+D)] or EER/CER.

Relative Risk Reduction	An estimate of the proportion of baseline risk that is removed as a result of the therapy. It is calculated as the ARR between the treatment and control groups divided by the absolute risk among patients in the control group or (CER-EER/CER).
Risk	The probability that an event will occur
Scientific Evidence	The product of well-designed and well-controlled research investigations that minimize sources of bias, considered the synthesis of all valid research studies that answer a specific question. The body of knowledge that has been derived from multiple studies investigating the same phenomena.
Secondary research	Filtered or synthesized publications of the primary research literature and include Systematic Reviews (SRs) or Meta-Analyses
Sensitivity	The proportion of *people with disease* or condition who *have a positive test* and is calculated using the formula a/(a+c).
Specificity	The proportion of *people free of a disease* who *have a negative test*, and can be determined using the formula d/(b+d).
Statistics	The branch of mathematics concerned with the collection, analysis, interpretation, presentation and organization of data so that they can be communicated in a meaningful way.
Statistical Significance	The likelihood that the results were unlikely to have occurred by chance at a specified probability level and that the differences would still exist each time the experiment was repeated. Therefore, statistical significance is reported as the probability related to chance, or "p" level
Synopsis or Critical Summaries	A *synopsis or critically appraised summary* of secondary (or primary) research is a 1-2 page critical summary of the SR/MA, or original research article plus an expert commentary. The commentary includes a critique of the strength and weakness of the methodology **and** of the evidence. The commentary concludes with the practical application of the research to practice along with any concerns or precautions.
Systematic Reviews	Summary of two or more primary research studies that have investigated the same specific phenomenon or question. This scientific technique defines a specific question to be answered, and uses explicit pre-defined criteria for retrieval of studies, assessment and synthesis of evidence from individual RCTs and other well-controlled methods. Methods used in SRs parallel those of RCTs in that each step is thoroughly documented and reproducible.
Treatment Effects	A comparison of the success rates of the experimental and the control treatment; provides a better estimate of treatment effects than p values alone and informs clinicians about the magnitude of treatment effects. An effect size is a statistical calculation that can be used to compare the efficacy of different agents by quantifying the size of the difference between treatments.
Therapy/Prevention Questions	Questions that look for answers that determine the effect of treatments that avoid adverse events, improve function and are worth the effort and cost.
Validity	The degree to which a study appropriately answers the question being asked or appropriately measures what it intends to measure.